Who says I can't?

A Guide to Living Well With COPD

To Diane

my "new, kind of normal", friend ☺

Joe x

Joe Lodge

© Joe Lodge 2015

First printed in this edition 2015

Joe Lodge has asserted his right under Section 77 of the Copyright, Designs and Patents Act 1988 to be identified as the author of this work.

All rights reserved. No part of this book may be reproduced, stored in a retrieval system, or transmitted in any form, or by any means, electronic, mechanical, photocopying, recording or otherwise without prior written permission from the author.

Requests to publish work from this book must be sent to Joe Lodge at duffersbook@outlook.com.

ISBN: 978-1-5196448-8-6

Book design: Dean Fetzer, www.gunboss.com

Disclaimer
This book is intended as an informational guide. The author is not medically trained and the contents of this book are the author's personal hints and tips based on his experience of COPD. Anyone trying any of the suggestions in this book should seek relevant medical or professional advice first. The author and publisher disclaim all liability and responsibility for any loss or injury that occurs directly or indirectly, due to the content of this book. The reader must take responsibility for the consequences of their own actions.

for Kim

Preface

I needed to write this book. I have always been a little outspoken and opinionated, but after having been diagnosed with COPD I realised that I felt the same as most patients, vulnerable and helpless. I couldn't accept those feelings without a fight. As I explored ways to get to grips with my new life, I met many patients along the way who were also struggling to deal with their condition. As time passed and I became physically and mentally stronger, I found that I was able to give them advice and encouragement. I think that it is comforting for someone who is feeling helpless to be offered a strong shoulder to lean on, so the idea of passing on my strength to as many people as possible was born. Write a book!

Planning to write a book and actually doing it are two completely different things of course. Where do I start? What do I want to say? What writing style will I adopt? Starting with my own early experiences was the platform upon which I built the book. If I could help people to at least challenge the way they felt now and the way they were managing their situation, and maybe improve it even a little, then my goal would be achieved.

What I could probably have written in six months was spread in fits and starts over nearly four years, as I dealt with a busy life trying to keep working, facing the challenges of being a lone parent and having many serious exacerbations that could distract me for months from any writing. I learnt to 'write when you're passionate, edit when you're not'.

As I tried to separate the book into three sections I would move a heading from one section to another, then back, or maybe it should really go here. Eventually, the headings started to take the form of a layout that began to appear almost book like. Nearly four years had passed since my journey began and now, suddenly, a book was appearing.

Then the mental analysis began. Will anyone like it? Will they find it useful? Have I done my best? As I had revealed some of my own personal life in the book, I also felt curiously exposed. But here I am, having tried to record in book form what I would be saying to you if we were sitting together with a coffee, discussing COPD.

So I finally present to you, the reader, my best of efforts to hopefully add to your knowledge and management of COPD with the sincere hope that you gain something from my words.

Acknowledgements

For assisting me during this journey I would like to acknowledge:

Liz Thompson, for inspiration and nudges during the 'doldrums'. "I still need nudging!"

Valerie Strawbridge for patient photographic assistance. "No more midge bites!"

Barry Carter for guiding me into the complicated world of book publishing. "Think I still owe you a coffee!"

Lesley Bell, for proof reading my manuscript and being the most sincere friend anyone could wish for throughout my journey. "Did I really have that many errors?"

Dean Fetzer of GunBoss Books for finally turning my manuscript into a printable format. "Thank goodness you understand bleed margins and pixels!"

All the staff on the Brearley Wing of the Northern General Hospital for patching me up time and again, always with a smile. "See you again sometime..."

Lastly, and most important of all, my daughter Kimberley who has patiently listened to my enthusiastic ideas and ramblings over the years, all the while appearing to be really interested! "Thanks..."

Many thanks to you all.

Contents

Introduction	1
Part 1 Diagnosis COPD	**5**
Diagnosis	7
Questions, questions	9
Bullet Holes and Shark Bites	11
Alpha 1 Antitrypsin Deficiency	15
What the hell happened?	16
So how long have I got...really?	17
Why me?	22
Depression	27
Pulmonary Rehabilitation Classes	28
Part 1 Summary	31
Part 2 Living with COPD	**33**
Getting the best from your inhalers	35
Get to know your body – Markers	38
Improve your strength and stamina	44
Oops...	62
Getting around – parking	63
Hospital	65
The Process	69
Ambulatory Oxygen	80
Self-Monitoring	85
Work	91
Shopping	94
Other medical issues	97
Stress and Emotions	98
Your Shrinking World	101

Partners	103
Cures	105
Trial Conclusion	114
Where do we go from here?	115
Part 2 Summary	118

Part 3 Enjoying life with Emphysema — 119

Enjoy life again	121
Find your passion	122
Micro Activity	126
Smart targets	145
Tai Chi Taster (Micro Tai Chi !)	148
Complementary Therapies	164
Supplements	168
The Other Passion	176
Reflections	177
Living with a 'duffer' – my daughter's perspective	180
Part 3 Summary	187

So what should I do next? — 189

Health Professionals	191
Friends	191
Family	192
Partners	193
You	194

Appendix A – Life Review Checklist — 197

Appendix B – Cure Trial Log — 201

About the Author

> "The man who says it can't be done should not interrupt the man who is doing it." Chinese proverb.

Introduction

I am a 'duffer'. As I write this book, I have lived with severe emphysema for fifteen years. I started out bewildered and scared that my life was suddenly going to deteriorate rapidly. How long was I going to live? How will I manage? How will my daughter cope? So many questions, and only vague answers that almost always began, "well, there are so many variables it's very difficult to say..."

Well I have survived this far, and managed as a lone parent. I have continued to work full time as a service manager in the electronics industry. I teach a Tai Chi evening class and look forward to a hike in the country whenever possible. I do everything for myself that it is possible to do. I have many interests and hobbies. Having to face the challenge of emphysema has forced me to review everything in my life and develop ways to achieve almost anything to the extent of my abilities. You can learn to 'be the best you can be', whatever level of disability you have.

Don't get me wrong, I still have days where I have to rest even after putting my socks on, days when it all goes out the window, but generally, I live life to the full. Most of this comes from understanding my mindset and the way this affects how I do everything, the way this changed after I was diagnosed, and how I developed a new mindset.

If you are reading this book, the chances are that you either have emphysema or another form of COPD, or you are a partner or relative of someone with COPD, or maybe you work with COPD patients. I hope whichever you are, you can gain some useful insight into what is possible when you learn to 'know yourself'. As I am not medically trained, these are just my personal experiences, observations, opinions, hints and tips. This book is intended as a guide to help you explore your changing mind-set and lifestyle as your COPD progresses.

The term 'duffer' that I use light heartedly to refer to myself is not the dictionary definition of 'stupid' but is based on the UK common usage of 'duff' as in "why do I always get the supermarket trolley with the duff wheel?" Duff is defined as 'not working properly', defective. I am a duffer.

The book is in three parts, Part One is about what happens when you are first diagnosed and have so many questions and so few, or definite, answers.

Part Two is about learning to cope with the available help for your condition.

Part Three is about making the transition from just coping to actually living with hopes, dreams, goals and enthusiasm like everyone else.

Who says I can't?

Remember, I have summarised fifteen years of experience in this book, so take your time reading it, or you may get out of breath! Of course, you will probably be somewhere along this path already, you will know where, as you read further. You may be far less breathless than I am and wonder what all the fuss is about, or you may be far worse and think that I have an easy life. Either way, I hope there is something here for you.

The whole point of this book is that you now find yourself with a life changing disease and you need to know many things about how to deal with it. My experiences are based on the UK system of care but as they mostly concern the mind-set, generally apply to anyone with COPD, anywhere.

Although I freely exchange the terms COPD and emphysema throughout the book to suit the context, I believe that the vast majority of it is also applicable to chronic bronchitis sufferers, who come under the same banner of 'obstructed breathing'.

Your health provider will arm you with a working knowledge of your disease, inhalers and medications, to manage daily issues and exacerbations, but if I can teach you one really important fact right now, it is that apart from this, the one thing that is going to make the **BIGGEST** difference to the rest of your life, is **YOU!** Join me on a journey into yourself and read on...

Part 1
Diagnosis COPD

Diagnosis

Having been an electronics engineer for most of my life, my working day was usually long and spent behind the wheel of the car travelling around the UK repairing various devices. As I was always under pressure to either get to the job on time or to get back home at some reasonable hour, 'proper meals' tended to go out of the window and would usually consist of snacks whilst driving. Crisps, chocolate and junk food would keep the hunger pangs at bay until the job was done and I could have a good meal later. Of course, many hours a day trapped in a car, having been a smoker of twenty years, did not help. Getting home late and tired would leave me 'past it', so proper meals often never really happened. Years of this must have had a detrimental effect on my health and contributed to my onset of emphysema. We all tend to battle on with life as it is, due to family and financial commitments, even when really we know it can't be good for us. I did plenty of that.

The truth is I had been getting more breathless on exertion for about a year prior to my diagnosis, and as all smokers do, I kept thinking that I should give up or at least cut down, then lit another cigarette while I pondered...

I had been struggling with what I thought was flu for a week or so, almost unable to breathe but struggling on to train a new engineer. I am an 'old school' engineer who is never off work unless completely incapacitated. Anyway, I ended up at home in a really bad way and my partner (now ex) called an ambulance. I spent the next three days in a high dependency unit. I had apparently got well developed pneumonia, severe dehydration, and was not in good shape at all. I remember a doctor sitting astride my chest and inserting tubes into my neck and I remember an airtight and horribly uncomfortable mask being put on my face which apparently forced oxygen into my lungs under greater pressure than the normal oxygen masks we are all familiar with, which I now understand to be a CPAP mask (Continuous Positive Air Pressure). It felt like I was in the scene from 'Alien' where a baby alien plants itself firmly on a man's face.

I was given intravenous antibiotics which eventually worked and I remained in hospital for some time until I had stabilised and improved. X-rays showed widespread damage to both lungs which was then diagnosed as emphysema. Further investigation and tests showed that I had genetic emphysema. I believe at this time my FEV1 (Forced Expiratory Volume) was 36% predicted (which means the amount of air you can breathe out in one second compared as a percentage to a healthy person of the same age, height and weight). I was told this was a pretty bad level to be diagnosed at. This is the first figure that we duffers learn, as it allows us to compare how bad we are. My observation is that when you meet patients with a similar FEV1 to your own, you subconsciously check whether they are better or worse than you at

Who says I can't?

handling it, or whether they are further down the 'slippery slope'. We always need to know how we fit in with others or the norm.

Questions, questions

I would bet money that the first questions that went through your head when you were first diagnosed and told that there is currently no cure for emphysema were, "how bad is it?", " how long have I got to live?", "can anything be done?"

The answer you received to the first question, "how bad is it?" was probably quite clinical and rightly so. Your x-rays and lung function tests provide pretty accurate information about the current status of your lung function. My x-rays showed widespread emphysema in both lungs and my FEV1 at 36% predicted simply means my lung function was about one third of a similar, healthy adult. My reaction to this was horror! "How the hell am I going to survive with only one third lung function?" Well, the latest FEV1 test I had, showed about 25% predicted. So here I am after fifteen years, not asking this question as often.

Now I don't get hung up on figures but just for perspective, if your FEV1 % predicted is above 40%, you have every opportunity to lead a very active life. Going from 36% to 25% as I have doesn't sound a massive drop, but if I still had 36% now, I would be trying to climb mountains, while at 25% I would be grateful to walk to the foot of a mountain! Even today, if I could improve my lung function by just 5% it would make a huge difference to what I can attempt or achieve. The lower your FEV1 % the greater the differential feels. Losing 5% at 50% would hardly be noticeable, but losing 5% at 25% would leave me 'grounded'.

The second question is the worst to come to terms with, "how long have I got to live?" Being diagnosed with a deteriorating, incurable disease is a massive blow that suddenly opens up all your raw feelings about life and death. It is being told that your life is going to be cut short. You may go into a state of panic or denial, that's natural. There are mental processes that you will have to go through to come to terms with what is happening. If you are newly diagnosed, the one piece of comfort I can give you is that maybe twenty years ago or more emphysema was a death sentence, but with modern medications it is likely you are going to live far, far longer than you think at this time. Emphysema has now become a chronic illness that may force you to dramatically change your lifestyle, but it is not the death sentence it used to be.

"Can anything be done?" When you first ask this question what you really want to hear is that it can be cured. At this time it can't. There are many trials and studies around the world and it is likely, as with all diseases today that some form of cure will eventually be found. However, we are not at that stage yet, and your health provider will give you various inhalers to keep the airways open, antibiotics for infections (your worst

Who says I can't?

enemy) and probably oral steroids to help reduce inflammation during infections (these also help you maintain better activity and appetite). They will probably recommend you to a pulmonary rehabilitation class (more of this later), to help you improve your physical health, which is likely to have deteriorated a lot by the time you get diagnosed. The class is for a set period, maybe six to eight weeks, followed by a 'maintenance' class. They will then recommend further activities and ways of managing your emphysema. This the first phase of learning to live with COPD.

At this stage your mindset is likely to be one of avoiding exertion and allowing others to do as much as possible for you, to help make life easier, while you come to terms with what is happening. This is correct, for now.

Bullet Holes and Shark Bites

Some months after my initial diagnosis, whilst learning to cope with my emphysema, I suddenly became almost unable to breathe at all. Once again an ambulance was called and a collapsed left lung was duly diagnosed. At the time I really thought it was the end. (When you're gasping for air and nothing's happening, like a fish out of water, this becomes a familiar feeling, but has been wrong up to now). Actually, looking back, the events following this are quite amusing (to me anyway), although they definitely were not at the time!

Joe Lodge

I was sitting upright in a chair so that the doctor could carry out the procedure to treat Pneumothorax (collapsed lung). This was to insert a needle with a tube connected, through the left side of my chest wall and into the lung lining to release the trapped air causing the lung to deflate. The doctor said that there aren't many pain receptors on the side of the body so it shouldn't hurt too much and, as it happened, he had a new American version of the needle that was much narrower than the English version and would like to give it a try. I believe I said "Yes, that sounds very interesting, I'm sure it would be beneficial for you at this time to be able to compare the differences between surgical appliances of various origins, however, I do feel that a little sense of urgency should prevail and I would really appreciate you commencing the procedure in the very near future." Or something along those lines, perhaps just a few short words...

The doctor duly inserted the implement, and to everyone's surprise, nothing happened. "That's unusual" said the doctor. "Yes it is, perhaps we could discuss that further..." I replied (No, not really....). So the good doctor followed with another attempt higher up this time. Same result! The doctor and I both tutted, even though I tutted whilst gasping for air. At this point I thought the lung was going to stay down followed quickly by myself. Anyway, common sense and a good old stiff upper lip later, the doctor returned with the wider English version, the 'Bulldog'. I was past caring, he could have put his left foot in my chest for all I cared, I just couldn't breathe! So

Who says I can't?

again, a little higher still, he inserted the British Bulldog...at which point, it felt like a bag of popcorn began to explode in my chest as air was filling my lung (the usable part anyway). Success! So to this day I am the proud bearer of three 'bullet holes' in my side (should be good for grandchild stories anyway). Obviously, the diameter of the insertion needle was not the issue, only the insertion point.

Perhaps it was difficult to judge as I have since learnt that with emphysema I have 'long' lungs due to the loss of elasticity, which also makes it difficult for x-ray operatives to get my lungs in the frame first time.

I don't know who was the most relieved, me or the doctor! He hid his feelings behind his professionalism. I don't know whether he was an experienced doctor or perhaps just exposed to the real job for the first time, which would be quite daunting. I didn't care anyway, as he completed the task. Doctors all have to learn along the way and I always try to be a model patient even when things don't go right. I have the greatest respect for everyone who has ever been involved in my treatment during the vast number of occasions I have been hospitalised. (I have to be nice, it's a small world...)

Over the years I have heard many people complaining about our hospitals but if they took a real look around the world they would see just how lucky we are in the UK. (And how much we complain!). Of course, over fifteen years of treatment, I have experience of and opinions about, not just doctors, but nurses, physiotherapists, support workers and just about everyone involved in healthcare. If you are a healthcare worker I must just say I really do love and respect you all, because no matter how overworked, understaffed or stressed you are, you always manage to patch me up and send me out 'fixed'.

Anyway, I digress. Following the lung inflation, a drain was left in my chest to ensure all the trapped air was expelled. That eventually happened, but there was still a trace of blood in the drain that wouldn't stop. Eventually I was told by a surgeon that he would have to perform a Thoracotomy (surgery to the lung). This would mean removing my left lung to investigate the bleed. This was done soon after, and they apparently discovered a large hole at the top of the lung which had not shown on the x-rays. After stapling the hole together and giving the lung lining a good dusting with talcum powder to ensure the resulting irritation would 'knit' the lung to the lining and prevent further deflations, all was well. So simple, so clever, and still going strong after fifteen years! ("Shhh, don't tempt fate!"). And you thought talcum powder was just for a baby's bottom!

There was just one further issue some couple of weeks after returning home, whilst the wound (a shark bite shape on my left back, another great feature for story telling!) was healing. One day. I was hit with the most piecing and agonising pain I have ever felt in my chest. It was so bad I almost couldn't breathe at all, and of course this was another ambulance and A & E visit. This happened a number of times in a few hours. It turned out that to remove my lung had meant cutting through some nerve fibres and as these had begun to knit back together they transmitted over zealous pain signals to my brain! Ouch!

A peculiar side effect I am going to share with you is that after the nerves had 'knitted' together and were working normally again, it became apparent that the front and back nerve fibres don't always connect to the corresponding ones, leaving me with a curious effect for many months...if I stroked the skin underneath my left nipple (now don't get giddy this is harmless!) I actually felt the sensation on my back, and vice versa. Anyway, the bottom line is that this lung has been fine ever since.

Following this, I then realised my life was going to be very different, it was explained, as before, that I had widespread emphysema in both lungs, which was also determined to be of genetic origin meaning I was always predisposed towards it and just had to supply the right triggers, which I appear to have done in abundance. I was booked in for follow up clinics and sent home, wondering what was going to happen now.

Alpha 1 Antitrypsin Deficiency

Don't worry if you can't pronounce it, it is just the technical term for genetic emphysema. Normally when your body detects a lung irritant or infection the white cells are despatched to engulf and destroy the intruder using enzymes called Neutrophil elastase. Once they have done their job, they are deactivated by a protein created in the liver called alpha-1 antitrypsin. Because of genetic emphysema, my liver hardly produces any of this, leaving the Neutrophil elastase to unwittingly continue to 'work'. This is a very powerful enzyme which will then start to destroy my own lung tissue, resulting in emphysema. This usually becomes apparent around the mid-forties but can cause problems at an earlier age. It is vital then that I use antibiotics as soon as I have an infection to minimise any damage my own body's defences will cause. Some patients with genetic emphysema go on to develop liver problems as well, but other than the self-damage and an occasional liver check-up, I have found very little difference in my condition to non-genetic emphysema patients. There is currently no cure for this deficiency although there are trials of augmentation therapy (to replace the deficiency) however the results are not yet conclusive enough for this to be available in the UK, so I have accepted what I have and get on with life.

What the hell happened?

There I was, one minute rushing headlong through life, meeting all the demands of a busy life and a family, trying to keep it all together, the next minute I was stopped in my tracks and told I had an incurable, progressive disease. I felt like curling into a foetal position and sucking my thumb. I just wanted someone to hug me and tell me it's all going to be alright. That didn't happen. My (then) partner was extremely concerned and family and friends were very sympathetic and supportive, but I realised that this was something I was going to have to come to terms with myself and I would have to dig deep to find ways of coping with it.

One thing I realised very quickly is that having emphysema (and most other chronic diseases) doesn't just affect you. It affects your partner, family and friends in many ways that change with time, not always for the better, and I hope that if they are reading this, I can help them to learn not only how best to support you now but how things will change in the future and how working together can prevent some pitfalls along the way.

So how long have I got...really?

Okay, let's tackle the BIG question. Your level of emphysema will have usually started to affect your lifestyle prior to diagnosis, causing you to seek help. Your diagnosis will have produced the x-rays and lung function results that allow the medical world to diagnose your severity of emphysema. Currently, the UK NICE (National Institution for Clinical Excellence) guidelines class my FEV1 of 25% predicted as Very Severe Emphysema. There, I am classified. Hey, this used to be called End Stage Emphysema which sounds terminal, so that's not so bad, is it?...hmm? This is what we need isn't it, always to know where we 'slot in'? To be able to compare how bad we are with others so we can see how long similar severities lived for. Hang on! It's not that simple, as you probably heard when you first asked your doctor this question. They will likely have said something quite vague about so many factors being involved it's almost impossible to predict your rate of decline or how long you will live.

It is quite possible for someone with very severe emphysema who doesn't smoke, exercises regularly and eats well, to outlive someone with mild emphysema who doesn't stop smoking, doesn't exercise and has a poor diet.

Once diagnosed, doctors will immediately tell you there are certain things that are vital towards prolonging your life, the most important being that if you smoke, STOP!

There is no question that if you continue to smoke you are shooting yourself in the foot and stopping is the single most important thing you can do to help yourself. No amount of medication is going to make much difference if you are going to continue smoking. I am not going to go on about this as you will hear it from everyone, especially in the early days of diagnosis. They are right and you know it. You will probably go through the mental phase of blaming yourself for not giving up before, but you can think of all those reasons why the time just wasn't right yet. Don't get me wrong, I smoked for twenty years before diagnosis and only finally kicked the habit after the three days in the high dependency

Who says I can't?

unit on forced oxygen and the following two weeks in a respiratory ward. Somehow that had enough mental impact to stop any further cravings. The threat of early death became my 'Sword of Damocles'. It probably helped that I had not been able to smoke while in hospital, giving me a head start. The habit was the hard part to deal with. Years before, I had tried hypnosis to stop smoking and amazingly, gave up instantly for about two years with no cravings, but life got difficult (divorce) and I somehow drifted back to smoking.

If I had needed help to stop after being diagnosed with emphysema I would have tackled it in a three pronged attack, which I had previously planned for many years, but never quite got around to. I would have tried the nicotine patches for the body's physical craving, along with hypnotherapy for the mental craving, adding dummy cigarettes (now electronic ones are available) for the habit. This would have worked for me. You have to try your own way, but I can tell you one thing, the thought of life without a cigarette may seem impossible when you smoke (that's just your subconscious helping you to stay in your comfort zone), but it is possible and you must try to find a way that works for you. Once you 'pop out' the other side of the craving phase, you will wonder why on earth you ever started in the first place. Everything is better, you can breathe easier, food is much tastier, and you don't smell like an old ashtray! Stop!

Anyway, the next factor that affects how quickly your lungs will decline is your medication. Not just the type of medication but how well you take it. Again, this is generally with short and long term inhalers to help keep your airways open, antibiotics for infections and steroids to reduce inflammation. There are other devices and products available that may help manage your emphysema, which your healthcare provider may recommend or you may find on the internet, we will look at these a little more, later.

Then of course, the next major factor is how you manage your body. Do you already have other medical conditions? How is your diet? How much exercise do you get normally? Was your glass half empty or half full before you were diagnosed? Are you depressed about your diagnosis? What were you doing with your life? All these things will have an effect on your rate of decline, as will your genetic predisposition (your likelihood of developing other issues or problems).

What about your environment? Do you still work? Do you ever get exposed to chemicals, smoke or dust? What is the background pollution level like in your local area? Do you or others use sprays or chemicals around the house? Do you have a dusty house? Carpets? Etc. etc. Think about all these factors and see if there is anything you can do to improve the negative ones.

Can you see where this is going? There are dozens of factors, some major, like smoking, some minor like how often you use public transport, but added together they will each have a very real effect on your daily condition and your long term quality of life and survival. Can you

Who says I can't?

begin to understand now why it is so hard for your doctor to predict how long you have to live? What needs to happen as you come to terms with your disease is for your mindset to change to ask a different question.

The correct question should really be "How long have I got to live if I do everything in my power to ensure the slowest possible decline in my lung function and maintain the maximum quality of life?" The correct answer in my opinion then becomes "Probably at least 70-80% of the normal predicted life span for your age at diagnosis, it's mostly down to YOU"!

I have a passion for all things scientific and technical and have spent many happy hours on the internet investigating all the technical aspects of emphysema and its treatment but in writing this book I wanted to address the real issue that has more effect than anything on your condition and that as I have just said, and will repeat many times is what YOU can do for YOU! All the facts and figures are available in other books and from your healthcare provider and the internet, so I have tried to keep these to a minimum, as I am trying to use my experience and knowledge to help you understand and guide your mindset.

Remember the saying, "You can lead a horse to water but you can't make it drink?" Well, you can provide a COPD patient with medications, knowledge and pulmonary rehabilitation, but you can't make them lead a healthy life style once you have set them off in the right direction. I think that there is a bit of a misconception by the medical world that because a patient has been diagnosed with COPD (or any other life threatening or changing disease) they will suddenly become very proactive in maintaining their health. Yes, of course they will initially, but then after time, when the system lets go of them, they may well slip back into whatever their natural mindset concerning health was, which, as with many people, is often of being complacent and not wanting to focus on 'good health' all the time just because you 'have to'.

Why me?

Once the dust settles and you have understood your diagnosis, been issued with inhalers and maybe booked on a rehabilitation course, things will probably start to sink in. You will no doubt go through the "why me" phase. "Could I have stopped this happening if I had lived a different lifestyle?" "I have been a good person, it's not fair this should happen to me." "I feel robbed of the rest of my life", "isn't there a magic bullet to make everything better?" and so on.

How you come to terms with all these thoughts and how they will affect you emotionally will depend on a number of things (here we go again). You may normally be of stout character and face things head on, or maybe your glass has always been half empty and this will leave you feeling pretty miserable. Maybe you're the anxious type and you will rip yourself apart with worry. You

Who says I can't?

might appear as the strong, cheerful type who is really panicking underneath but tries to put a brave face on. You may just get on with dealing with it.

How you view this attack on your lifespan will also depend on your beliefs. You may be very religious and see this as God's will (your own God, whatever your religion). Maybe you question your God. Maybe you're an atheist who doesn't have or need anyone to question or blame. Maybe you believe in karma and see it as 'payback'. Perhaps, like me you have genetic emphysema, passed on by your parents. Is it their fault? Is it your Grandparents fault? Is it just the way things are? So many possibilities.

Whatever your beliefs, it has happened, and you have to deal with it. You can blame life for dealing you a bum card, you can curse yourself for doing wrong in a previous life or leading an unhealthy lifestyle in this one. You can think so many things and end up feeling quite sorry for yourself even if you don't admit it. I guess I am one of the lucky ones as I have always been a positive person, so having to overcome a few challenges is all part of the rich tapestry of life. If life was all rainbows, I wouldn't grow in spirit (the human spirit that is, I am not religious but do believe the human race should continually strive to improve itself).

It is how it is, and you have the choice to spend the rest of your life as a victim, or grab it by the horns and make the most of it.

Joe Lodge

If you really are finding it hard to feel any control over your COPD, let me address two issues.

First, the feeling of self-pity, **'poor me'**. You need to get this in perspective. You are going to have to change your lifestyle and find new ways to tackle things. That's not so bad. At this time you are probably getting all the sympathy you could wish for from your partner, family and friends and that's really important in the early stages, but, if you're not careful, this can change with time which I will return to in a later chapter. The trouble with sympathy is, it just keeps feeding the flame, and it doesn't actually help you or make any change to your life. It just strokes the inner child.

Try this if you don't agree. Ask all your family and friends to gather at your house and sit in a big circle with you at the centre. Ask them all to focus completely on you for fifteen minutes and give you non-stop, intensive sympathy, whilst you feel as sorry for yourself as possible. Then stop and see how much difference this has made to how you really feel inside. Let me guess, none whatsoever, other than possibly leaving you feeling a little sheepish. It's just not a constructive way forward, so maybe it's time to let this feeling go.

Now ask them to each take a turn saying all the funny or sarcastic things they can think of about you and your emphysema like "you're just having a bad 'air' day" or "can you just blow up this balloon?" or maybe "can you just blow into this breathalyser please sir?" (Ha! Picture

Who says I can't?

that one!). Now see who ends up smiling and feeling better. (You...and your partner, family and friends?).

Do yourself a favour and swap sympathy for light hearted sarcasm any day, it's so much more fun and will help you and those around you deal with your emphysema without becoming morbid. Go on, really try it, I dare you!

If that doesn't work then I suspect you really are a serious person, so here's another angle for you to consider. Whilst writing this book and almost by complete chance I came across a book called Breathe by James Fordham. It has nothing whatsoever to do with COPD but is a cancer survivor's story in diary form of how he faced and overcame the challenges ahead. What really struck me and the reason I mention it, is that I realised that cancer is a very urgent, aggressive and unpredictable beast, in complete contrast to COPD, which is slow, insidious and comparatively predictable. It made me realise how lucky I was to have my C word rather than his C word. I have plenty of time to think about how to deal with my COPD, plenty of time to find interesting ways to stay active and plenty of time to plan ahead for the darker days. I actually felt very lucky after reading this book. If you really can't get to grips with having COPD, I would recommend you read it and get your situation in perspective.

The second issue is, "how are you today?", "well, not so good really, I've been coughing a lot and don't think I will manage the shopping trip, my breathing is rubbish today and I feel really weak." "Oh dear, well I hope you feel better tomorrow, gosh is that the time, must dash."

Joe Lodge

"How are you today?" "Well still not so good"...this is how it is going to go...forever! Stop it, people are genuinely interested and all love and care for you but will eventually get fed up hearing the same old lines and you will become a grumpy old sod. Try finding an obviously incorrect statement that at least brings a smile to both your faces. My stock reply to that question, no matter who asks or how bad I am (unless it's a serious doctor), is "Wonderful" with a big smile! Yes we both know its waffle, I have emphysema, but at least it saves us both going down the sad path and we both smile. Try it for a day.

Those of you around in the seventies may remember hearing about Emile Coue, who was quoted by an Australian broadcaster. Each morning on his radio show, he asked listeners to repeat with him, "Every day, in every way, I am feeling better and better." So many people reported positive feelings after doing this for a while. The power of suggestion? Self-deception? It doesn't matter if it works. If you keep telling yourself positive things eventually they will become the norm for you. Try it.

Pay careful attention to your speech. Every time you say "I used to be able to...", "I can't do that now", "I wouldn't even be able to attempt that", you are reinforcing your subconscious, negative approach to life. Try to catch yourself and just think about what you are saying or about to say, then try to substitute positive statements like, "I'm going to try", "I'm going to see if I can find a way to do that at my pace", "I think it would be fun to have a go!". Reprogram yourself!

Who says I can't?

Depression

No matter what medication or support you have for your lungs, it will not help if you slide into depression. I think it is common for any patient with a chronic illness to potentially suffer depression and I know many on further medications like Prozac. Although I am naturally positive and will always look for solutions to any problem, there have been times where I have noticed my thoughts becoming more negative, especially when I have been in hospital with pneumonia and then spent months recovering. After a long period, even I start to think that my breathing has now gone down another notch and this is the way it will be. "Will I be able to keep working?" "Will I ever do my Tai Chi again?" "Can I keep going long enough to get my daughter through university?"

Every single time, there has been one thing that has started me on the road to avoiding depression...ACTION! Getting up and doing something. Stop sitting at home feeling sorry for yourself and take one small step. Go and buy a new plant or visit the zoo with your grand-kids. It doesn't matter so long as you **stop thinking and start doing**. Activity releases 'feel good' chemicals in the brain. There's a time to think and a time to 'do'.

Think when you are feeling positive, act when you are feeling negative!

Joe Lodge

Pulmonary Rehabilitation Classes

I believe most people in developed countries have access to these and they are probably the first real positive thing that happens after diagnosis. I remember going to my first assessment. After a number of tests and adjustments to the figures to compensate for my age, height and weight, the nurse informed me I had an equivalent lung age of 113! Now I was having a good day up to then, 113! But I'm only 40 something! I can only guess what equivalent age my lungs are now, so no birthday candles for them.

The actual classes, done over say, a six week period, consist of a number of simple exercises designed to increase your strength and stamina in a controlled environment. Pulmonary rehabilitation classes are also interesting as they bring in various experts to discuss your breathing, diet, exercise etc. You must realise that Pulmonary Rehabilitation is not an end in itself but a beginning. **It's what you do with the improved strength and stamina afterwards that will make all the difference.** You may be encouraged to join a gym which could help maintain your level of fitness or join a Breathe Easy group of similar patients, for group activities.

Whatever happens after this point will be down to you!

Who says I can't?

Just a note for those who run the Pulmonary Rehabilitation classes. I was lucky when I attended classes as they were run by COPD nurses often with a wicked sense of humour and the classes were fun and motivated. I understand that currently some classes are now outsourced and may have the brief that patients 'need' to do this for their benefit. Whilst that may be true, the class **MUST** be fun! While the exercises alone may be clinically proven to improve strength and stamina whether or not it's fun and light hearted, the mental association for the patient will be either something they really enjoyed, had a good laugh at and can't wait for the next class, or something serious that they are expected to attend because they 'should want to get better'.

Which subconscious association do you think will help to give them the positive mindset and motivation in the future when they think about activity?

You have a tremendous responsibility running a Pulmonary Rehabilitation class. This may be the final and lasting experience many patients have of the 'system' before they are released to find their own way forward. Having a 'boot camp' experience of being continually told you can do better does not help. It is incredibly hard to get your body going when you just can't breathe. Imagine placing a plastic bag over your head with a few pinholes in it. Would you be eager to try doing the exercises? It is not simply about will power. The patients will often start the class feeling very vulnerable. They are about to expose their limits, physically, mentally and emotionally, and you need to be empathetic to this in the way you communicate with and encourage them, as how you do this can have a huge and long lasting effect on their future approach to activity. Just because they are ill doesn't mean they don't still have pride. Treat them as you would want your parents to be treated; encourage and push them with a smile, and everyone goes home happy. Make your class the one everyone wants to attend! Thank you.

Take exercise seriously but don't do it seriously!

Who says I can't?

Part 1 Summary

- The one thing that is going to make the BIGGEST difference to the rest of your life is YOU!

- If you smoke, STOP! FULL STOP!!

- Swap sympathy for light hearted sarcasm!

- Think when you are feeling positive, act when you are feeling negative.

- Pulmonary Rehabilitation classes are a great launch pad, whether you reach for the stars or not is down to you!

- Take exercise seriously but don't do it seriously, it MUST be fun!

Part 2
Living with COPD

Getting the best from your inhalers

The most useful daily tools you will use are your inhalers. Don't waste them! Each time you use them, remember you want to get the spray as deep as possible into your lungs. What can you do to ensure you get the maximum effect every time? Start by preparing your lungs. If you are huffing and puffing, just allow yourself to wait a few minutes until you can be a little more relaxed and settle your breathing (unless you are using them for an asthma attack) otherwise you will take very weak, shallow breaths, which are not going to carry the spray very deep, or you will be puffing it out before it even gets fully in…slow down and relax before you take your inhalers.

Next, clear your lungs of stale air and get the diaphragm working. Sit or stand comfortably, but upright. Exhale as far as you can then pause, exhale some more, keep doing this as long as possible until you feel your stomach really 'screwed up' pushing the diaphragm up. Then relax the stomach and shoulders and allow yourself to inhale comfortably and fully. Repeat this a few times until your lungs feel clear and your diaphragm is 'ready for action'.

If you take a fast acting inhaler, such as Ventolin (Salbutamol, blue inhaler), my personal thought is that it makes sense to take this before any longer acting inhaler, such as Atrovent (Ipatropium Bromide, green inhaler). I take the Ventolin first, then wait a few minutes, as this opens the airways very quickly, improving the chances of the longer acting inhaler penetrating deeper into the lungs. If you use a spacer, don't be complacent. You will probably have been instructed to breathe normally after squirting the inhaler into the spacer. This is fine so long as 'normally' is a reasonably deep breath. If you can, take a slight pause after each inhalation, to give the spray a chance to adhere to the lung lining, before you exhale. Also, try to exhale very gently so as not to blow the spray straight back out.

Whether you use a spacer or not, I have found it more effective, just before you begin to inhale, to lean slightly forward as you exhale, helping to squeeze the stale air out of the lungs, then stay upright or lean very slightly back as you inhale. Experiment for yourself which method leaves your airways feeling most open. Bear in mind the depth and effectiveness you achieve can vary depending on the temperature (we all know what cold air does to the airways!) and your current lung status (clear, phlegmy, tight) as well as your inhalations.

If you use a steroid inhaler as well (I currently use the Seretide 500 Accuhaler), this is likely to be of the micro-powder type. I wait for at least 20 minutes after taking the 'opening' inhalers before taking this, to allow the best chance of deep inhalation. Again, try for a short pause after inhaling to allow the powder to stick.

When I am out and about, I do not always carry my spacer, so I have to pay special attention to inhaling correctly. As I am going to spray the inhaler directly into

Who says I can't?

my mouth, I need to ensure that the force of air I am inhaling is stronger than the force of the spray, otherwise I will just be spraying it at the back of my throat. Being accomplished at abdominal breathing, I don't have a problem with this, I just need to ensure that my inhale is as powerful as possible by really working the diaphragm and by timing the squirt just **after** I begin inhaling, so a really strong air current carries the spray down into the lungs without it hitting the back of my throat. It is not difficult to learn with a bit of practice and careful attention. I have seen so many people using inhalers like breath fresheners, just a couple of quick squirts into the mouth. I always wonder how they get any benefit at all.

One other point about inhalers that people sometimes forget is that they are a liquid until sprayed. To give them the best chance of creating a fine mist, they need to be shaken, vigorously if possible a few times before use. If I am using them outdoors, in the car, or anywhere where they have become cold, I also warm them in my hands for a minute, with my thumb on the metal top, to help them vaporise better. You may find it embarrassing using inhalers in public, but there are many tricks to help like pretending you're looking in a shop window or waiting until there is a noise to use the spray so you don't draw attention to yourself. I have to give you a warning though...I was sitting in the car one day, parked with my side of the car nearest the pavement. I was waiting for my daughter, who had popped into a shop. As we would not be home for a while and it was time for my inhalers, I thought I would take the opportunity. Now if you have shaken an inhaler at chest height you know it looks pretty silly and draws attention to you, so, I innocently decided to shake it down under the steering wheel, out of site. Just as I was doing this, a man was walking past the car from the front to the rear, and he was looking at me. As our eyes met he immediately looked away and I instantly realised why (think about it!). Did I die of embarrassment? Yes! But at least I lived to tell the tale and learnt the lesson. Now I am quite happy to shake my sprays in full view of the public!

Get to know your body – Markers

This is so important. There are a number of small routines you perform daily, no matter how simple or subtle, that can become your 'yardsticks' if you pay attention to them. You can then use them to note the effects of a whole manner of things, exercise, medications, infections, supplements etc. It is a very useful tool if you spend the time paying attention to how you feel and breathe normally when doing these things, until it is second nature. The more 'tuned in' you become, the more sensitive you will become to noticing even slight changes. As your emphysema is unlikely to go away (No, really, it's not) you should get smart and arm yourself with all the tools you can to make life easier!

Who says I can't?

Depending on your life and routines, your markers may be different from mine, but they are easy to identify and quantify. Here are mine:

Getting dressed

This is the first thing I do each day (well actually the second, the first is to wake up, but unless I have an infection, my breathing is usually reasonable at this point). You may put on a dressing gown. I get dressed. The hardest part I find is putting on socks. "Well don't then, put your slippers on!" you may say, but I need to put my socks on. As I have done it so many times, I can tell the slightest change in how out of breathe I am. The reason for this is because I have to 'scrunch up' leaning forwards and down, which is not ideal for breathing. That is my first marker of the day.

Washing/shower

My preference is to take a shower rather than a bath. I have not had many baths and no, I am not smelly, it's because I find a bath is usually too hot and if I only run warm water it is just as uncomfortable and feels cold. The whole body is immersed in the hot water, which draws blood to the skin, as you know because it reddens. I find this increases the work needed by my lungs, just as digestion after a heavy meal does, affecting my breathing.

Also, I have to sit and 'scrunch up' in a bath, again not conducive towards breathing.

Give me a shower any time. You can stand comfortably, or if not strong enough or during a bad 'air' day, you can put a plastic chair in the shower and sit on that. I don't have the shower too hot. Washing my hair and applying shower gel are very definite markers, as any reduction in breathing makes this extremely difficult. When I have an infection it is usually just too much effort to have a shower (then I probably do smell but everyone is so polite, hey?). Anyone with my level of emphysema will know exactly what I mean. Getting dried afterwards can also be daunting. The best way I have found is to use a hooded bathrobe. I can just slip into this and dry slowly without feeling cold and without any effort, although I always try to use a towel if possible, following the premise of maintaining as much activity as possible. It is sometimes difficult but is another little 'workout' that I could easily miss. Realistically, as I have to get ready for work in the morning, I would leave showering for the evening when I have more time.

Exercise – Tai Chi

I am lucky to have discovered Tai Chi soon after my diagnosis. As you may know, this is a series of gentle, flowing movements, performed daily in the same way. I always wait until after I have had my first daily inhalers, to get the best possible benefits. As I am so familiar with the movements, I can again tell instantly where on the scale of breathing and 'wellness' I am. I say 'wellness' as again, anyone with emphysema will know, not only do you have bad 'air' days for no apparent reason, but also days when you just don't feel well. Markers help you know where on the scale you are.

Eating

Depending on how good or bad my breathing is, eating and breathing at the same time can feel very difficult. It sounds funny when you say it, but eating can be quite exhausting. It's important to chew your food as much as possible to give your stomach less work to do and hopefully not impact on your breathing, but at the same time, chewing can become tiring. If I am ill at all I will try to use easy to eat foods like scrambled eggs. Try not to lose your appetite as this will compromise your immune system. When I have been really weak I have even considered (but not dared to try...yet) using the blender on say, a Sunday Lunch (beef, potatoes, vegetables, Yorkshire pudding, gravy)...yummy! (Of course that would be if someone else cooked it. Luxury!)

Walking/inclines

You will definitely get to know your good day 'norm' and your bad day 'norm'. It is easy to spot any variation in this if you pay attention. Even the slightest incline can be hard work, depending on your breathing at the time. This is probably the most obvious of markers. It is surprising that you will be aware of inclines in say, a shopping mall that 'normal' people didn't even register. As a marker this only applies to an incline you use every day though.

Which side is easier to lie on

Sleeping on the back is usually a 'no go' area for me, as I soon begin to feel like I am drowning. I usually start on my right side until I wake up, then change to my left. If I wake a number of times in the night, I will change sides each time so my lungs don't become lopsided, where one side is relaxed and does most of the work while the other side is compressed and becomes weaker. I try to balance the workload to keep both sides as active as possible. I believe that anatomically it is easier on the lungs to sleep on the right hand side due to the position of the heart in relation to the lungs. The trick is to pay attention to how it feels to you, so as well as being a marker, you can also get the most benefit from your sleep.

Bad 'air' days

These just happen. You may be feeling fine one day and even plan a good day out for tomorrow, only to wake up just unable to breathe. You do not feel ill as if you had an infection, and you did not overdo it the day before. You may have been eating and sleeping well. You may be able to pin it down to something but most likely you

Who says I can't?

won't. It is one of those days. It may be frustrating for you and even more so for your partner, family or friends if you planned to do something together, but you (and they) have to learn to just accept it happens. No amount of grumbling at you or coercing (it is not about will power) will change it. Better to always assume this can happen and plan accordingly. The point is you may not be able to quantify it, so unless the cause is obvious, don't try.

In the early days of my emphysema I religiously monitored and recorded everything! Outside temperature, air pressure, humidity, pollen count, exposure to hairsprays and deodorants, meals and so on. I have never yet managed to identify anything that consistently causes bad 'air' days (except smoke of course!), so now I don't bother and just go with the flow. Of course, I try to avoid any extremes like high temperatures, pouring rain and freezing winds. (Update. I do find now at 25% FEV1 that the weather does make my breathing more difficult on days where there 'is no air').

Learn to pay attention to these or other markers, so that you can use them as a measuring tool. The effects of a new or changed medication can be judged against your normal markers. The benefits of any supplements or exercise can also be judged. Foods that help or hinder can be identified. Markers can help towards you feeling you have some control over what is happening to you.

Markers 'rock'...listen to your body.

Joe Lodge

Improve your strength and stamina

As your emphysema progresses and you are less able to do normal activities, both your strength and stamina will decrease. This is not the way forward. As you do less work with your upper limbs especially, the muscles weaken and waste. This is one of the indicators of your remaining time. You may have done Pulmonary Rehabilitation and managed to use some weights to maintain or improve your strength and stamina, however, unless you maintain this afterwards they will gradually decline again. Now, it's okay recommending that you attend the gym to keep strong and fit, but in my observations, the gym is mostly full of pretty fit people who enjoy working out and just want to get fitter. Then there are those who 'need' to visit the gym to lose weight or get fit for medical reasons. For most of us, especially those advised to attend for health reasons, it's difficult to maintain the passion. Indeed, most health professionals I know are the worst offenders when it comes to exercise! Doing something because you 'have to' doesn't last.

I know it is important for me to maintain and improve my muscle strength but going to the gym is so time consuming. Travel, parking, changing, all take time and effort, "maybe I'll give it a miss today". Having a busy lifestyle, I needed to bring the gym to me so I was more likely to make the effort. I find it hard to do exercise that involves both arms and legs together. I love to row boats

Who says I can't?

and find the position of slightly leaning forward very comfortable for breathing. This allows my shoulders and arm muscles to have a really good session without needing any will power as I am just playing. I was going to get a rowing machine to use at home during winter but they take up so much room. I have found the answer in just a simple, rubber, rowing device. It has a stirrup for each foot, then about a metre of rubber splitting to two handles. I can just row to my heart's content even watching TV, so it doesn't become boring, and then simply store it in a drawer. £10 well spent! (Just type rowing and rubber on Amazon...never just type rubber on Amazon unless you like dressing up!)

For my legs I really enjoy cycling. I discovered that I can cycle easier and farther than I can walk. Again I think this is due to the slight forward lean and not using as many muscles as walking to maintain posture etc. You may be lucky enough to have your own bike, I usually hire one at a nearby country park, so I can enjoy the cycle without paying much attention to the actual exercise. In the future I may buy one as there are now folding mountain bikes available which you can easily leave in the car boot. During winter it is obviously too cold to cycle (for me), so I was looking at exercise cycles. Again, they take up so much room. I was thinking that I only needed it for my legs and there are some simple models available that are just the base with pedals. I have bought one of these and find that if I sit on the sofa arm as my saddle, I can peddle away happily while watching TV, and the unit easily stows away behind the sofa. (mini exercise cycle on Amazon). Oops, I'm beginning to sound like a bit of a TV addict here! I usually select a good music channel to cycle to and crank up the volume. The point is it's easy to make exercise just a bit of fun if you think about it, and **exercise MUST be fun** if you are to maintain it!

I find that stamina is stored in the muscles. The more activity you do, the more you can do and the more you want to do. You will find if you go through periods of illness when you just can't exercise, that when you feel well enough again, you have lost all your stamina. I just begin again, gently, and allow my body to strengthen slowly.

Upper limbs

As I mentioned previously, you may not be aware but one of the indicators of morbidity (how far down the slippery slope you are) is how thick your arms are. The chances are, if you have been in any group of people with COPD you will be familiar with the arms getting thinner and thinner. With that in mind I intend to keep my arms as strong as possible. The problem is, as your breathing deteriorates over the years you take on less and less everyday jobs that would normally keep your muscles toned.

If my arms have become really weak, usually after an exacerbation, where I may have done no exercise for possibly weeks, I start with a Powerball. You can find these very cheaply on the internet (Amazon again, wish I

Who says I can't?

got commission!). It is a ball shaped object about the size of a tennis ball, made of plastic, with a spinning inner part that forms a gyroscope. The simple version uses a pull string to start the inner spinning, the more expensive versions have a battery start. The idea is to hold the ball and rotate the wrists or arms in various positions, working different arm muscles. It is a strange feeling as the ball tries to prevent the movement due to the gyroscope effect. The outcome is that you are moving your arms against a resistance, building both strength and stamina in a relatively gentle way. This is the lowest level arm exercise I have used so far, so it is a good starting point. As my strength and stamina increase I try to use body building hand dumbbells to build muscle. The Powerball is then great to warm the muscles followed by groups of slow curls with the dumbbells to build strength.

Again, if you pay attention to what you are doing at all times, you will find many small, daily opportunities that you may have avoided previously, to help maintain arm strength, like carrying the shopping bags instead of letting the family help. When using a watering can in the garden, instead of a hose, as I fill the watering can, I have an opportunity to raise the can a number of times in each arm before actually emptying it (when I am well and strong enough of course!).

Simply paying attention and making a small effort can help reduce the deterioration of your arm bulk and leave you feeling empowered that you are doing something positive and helping to slow your demise...great stuff!!

Joe Lodge

Breathing

Breathing is something you have done without thinking all your life and now it doesn't function as well as you would like, you will have to learn to take some conscious control of it. There are two types of breathing you will be taught as an emphysema patient, abdominal breathing and pursed lip breathing. Generally, abdominal breathing will be the normal, relaxed breathing pattern to use for rest or gentle activities, while pursed lip breathing is needed for exertion. Ideally you should always inhale through the nose to warm the air and trap particles, however, as emphysema progresses this becomes more difficult.

You do not need to get technical about how your lungs work, but you must always remember one important fact, they aren't just for breathing in oxygen, they are for the exchange of gases. Oxygen is inhaled as it is needed by every cell in your body to function properly, but just as important is carbon dioxide, the waste product of your cell's activities. Your body must not just get rid of carbon dioxide, but maintain a proportional balance between inhaled oxygen and exhaled carbon dioxide. This is something you are probably acutely aware of already but may not have thought about. If you have emphysema and you try to walk briskly, compared to your normal pace, without altering your breathing, you will very quickly grind to a halt and feel like you are going to seize up, not because

Who says I can't?

you can't breathe in but because your body feels physically terrible. You will know this feeling. This isn't just from a lack of oxygen, it is the build-up of carbon dioxide as your lungs are not able to exhale it efficiently enough. The purpose of pursed lip breathing is to help you gain more control over this kind of scenario.

Normally, to inhale, your diaphragm muscle (like a rubber sheet stretched across the abdomen below the rib cage) will relax and sink down, expanding the lung volume thereby creating a vacuum which draws air in. To exhale, the diaphragm is contracted and as the lungs are elastic they shrink again, forcing air out. With emphysema, the lungs lose their elasticity, making correct exhalation difficult. Your body will try to compensate by making the diaphragm, the rib muscles (intercostal) and neck muscles work harder to help maintain the status quo. The trick when learning to take more conscious control over your breathing is to strengthen these muscles and use them more efficiently.

Cleansing Breath

Now all this talk about learning abdominal and pursed lip breathing is all well and good, as you will then be drawing fresh oxygen in as deep as possible to your lungs, and ridding them of carbon dioxide. However, as you have emphysema, you are not very good at expelling air, so the chances are there is still a lot of stagnant air in the dark corners of your lungs. So, before you begin any breathing exercises, it is worth spending a couple of minutes clearing out as much of the stagnant air from the lungs as possible. Let's call this Cleansing Breathe.

Sit or stand as you will for your breathing exercise. Now begin by just blowing out as much air as you can for as long as you can, comfortably, then a little more. Notice on that last push how your stomach muscles tense. Now allow your stomach to relax and open your arms wide as you take a big breathe in through the mouth. Now, again, begin to blow out as much as you can for as long as you can, but at the same time slowly lean forward and cross your arms in front of you, as though your left hand was trying to reach your right knee, and you right hand was trying to reach your left knee. This action helps to 'squeeze' the lungs and get all that stale air out. Repeat this four or five times, then relax and breathe normally. That's done it gently, now a little more vigorously. Now, taking a normal breath in, blow out again but not in one go. Break it into say five blows out. Then another slow breath in. Maybe you can only manage two or three, maybe six or seven. It doesn't matter, it is all helping to 'work' your lungs and clear stagnant air.

The most effective technique for a cleansing breath I have found over the years, is to use many short sharp blows to the tune of a common English football chant often heard at matches. I can only describe it as blow blow – blow blow blow – blow blow blow blow – blow blow – the last two blows usually include the team's

Who says I can't?

name. Now I don't pretend to be a follower of the good game so I am not expert in what this may be called, but whenever a match is being played, the fans will clap their hands to this tune followed by chanting the team's name. I understand this is actually based on a 1962 song by the Routers called 'Let Go (Pony)' easily found on the internet. Try doing this three times continuously, it really loosens the diaphragm! Practice. Find the best way for you to clear your lungs of stale air. Clear out the 'cobwebs' before you begin breathing practice. It is a really smart move to do this before using inhalers, so that they get the best chance of being inhaled deeply into the lungs.

Astute readers may ask the question, "How on earth did you discover and use that chant for your breathing?" My response would be, "That's a very good question, well-constructed and presented, and I'm really pleased you asked me that, it shows you are paying attention, now, moving on..."

Abdominal Breathing

If you have not learnt this yet, it is a real skill that may take a while to master, but will pay handsome dividends! Most healthy people are shallow breathers to start with, where does that leave you when you get emphysema? Breathless, to say the least. Are you a shallow breather? Try this. Sit or stand comfortably and just relax for a minute so that your breathing is normal for you. Now place your left hand gently on your abdomen and your right hand gently on your chest. Without taking any control, just pay attention to the movement of the hands. Which hand appears to be moving most? It's usually the chest hand but well done if it's the abdomen hand. What you need to try to achieve at rest or during very light activity (how light will depend on the severity of your emphysema) is to get maximum movement of the hand on your abdomen. When you do this, you are getting maximum travel from your diaphragm allowing air to be drawn much deeper into the lungs. You need to learn to both relax and strengthen the diaphragm muscles.

Now relax your arms by your side if standing and on your lap if sitting. Just breathe normally but now start to pay attention to your breathing. Start to gently breathe in through the nose and out through the mouth. As abdominal breathing is a very good form of relaxation exercise it is worth spending a little time each day to practice this. If your breathing is so bad you can't inhale through the nose, then just inhale through the mouth. Everything you do must be at a level comfortable for you. Now imaging there is a balloon in your stomach which is connected by a tube to your nose. Each time you inhale through your nose, relax your stomach and allow the balloon to inflate, as you exhale, gently squeeze your stomach muscles helping to empty the balloon. Don't rush or force your breathing, just allow this to develop slowly and consistently. Once you get the hang of it, it will help you to feel calm and relaxed after just minutes.

Who says I can't?

In through the nose, out through the mouth. Practice this for a few minutes. If you find you are struggling for air or feel light headed, just stop and breathe normally, you are probably trying too hard and have not got the right balance yet between inhale and exhale.

The timing of inhale and exhale is something you may never have considered before, as to most people it is an unconscious change that the body just takes care of. Remember when you used to run to catch that bus? You didn't think "I need to increase my breathing now", it just happened. Now life is different and you need to learn to pay attention to how you should be breathing during different activities. Usually with abdominal breathing while you are relaxed, you will find it more comfortable to have longer out breaths than in breaths. Try varying these gently by counting seconds and get to know what is normal and comfortable for you. Maybe start counting slowly to three for the inhale and to five for the exhale to start with. With regular practice you will learn to become more sensitive to your normal breathing, and then, the effects of not breathing in and out in the right ratio will be more obvious and, depending on your activity, you can quickly adjust.

A tip. As you are going to have to learn to have greater control over your diaphragm muscles, it is as well to practice strengthening exercises. Regular deep breathing will help strengthen the diaphragm. An additional aid to this (especially if you're lazy!) is to get yourself a rubber hot water bottle. Fill it with warm water (not hot). Lay on the floor or bed while maybe watching TV (oops, there I go again!) or reading a book, and place the bottle on your stomach, then just practice gentle abdominal breathing. The diaphragm muscles now have to work a little harder which will help strengthen them over time. You know the key to relaxation, breathing and strengthening exercises is a little every day. Don't try marathon sessions, they will either exhaust you or overwork the muscles.

Abdominal breathing can become the norm if you consciously practice it daily and always try to be mindful of how you are breathing. Think how much your body will appreciate the extra oxygen, allowing you and your internal organs to feel so much more relaxed.

Pursed lip breathing

While abdominal breathing is good for all normal activity where you can manage it, it is no use when you are breathless, during or after exertion. You will no doubt be very aware of the effect of climbing stairs. Depending on how severe your breathing is you may make it to the top and feel like collapsing or maybe you only get up a stair or two at a time. What you need to learn is one simple lesson....during activity, forget about breathing in...JUST BREATHE OUT! This is the most important breathing lesson. When you feel like you are going to seize up it is because your carbon dioxide level is too high and you need to get rid! Blow out. Inhaling will happen on its own

Who says I can't?

if you just focus on exhaling. Exhale through pursed lips, just as you would to blow out a candle flame.

Before you try any breathing techniques on the stairs, just try this. Walk briskly as far as you can normally, just breathing however you have up to now. Make a note of how far you get before you have to stop. Now do the same again but consciously count your in and out breaths. Start by saying in or out on each step, try OUT OUT OUT IN OUT OUT OUT IN ie. three exhales to each inhale. You may find you need to increase the exhales to four or five and the inhales to maybe two or three, depending on your level of emphysema and the pace you are walking at. Don't rush this, it is an individual thing you have to learn to adjust for your particular level of severity. You can learn to match different walking paces and different in /out ratios to do different things.

I remember when I first became a lone parent. It was not planned in advance and I had to give up my full time job. My daughter was eight at the time. I had worked loyally for my company for a number of years and asked them if I could keep my company car for a few weeks until I sorted a car out. With my emphysema I would be lost without a car. They said no. I guess I still haven't forgiven them for that. Anyway, my daughter's school was a good mile away. I was going to have to get her there and back (and myself!) each day. There were buses, but we lived in between stops. The nearest stop was in the wrong direction, easier to walk to but if I miss the bus then I have further to walk! If I wait at the bus stop that is in the right direction and I'm too late, I won't be able to rush to school before the bell goes! If I see the bus coming, I can't run for it! "Grrr!" Welcome to the world of emphysema! This is why our world shrinks. Any kind of travel always brings the same, 'what if' nightmares.

Anyway, I had no choice but to make sure I got to school on time whether the buses ran to timetable or not, and as I could never be sure about the buses, or the weather, or my level of breathing, I decided I had to find a way to 'power walk' there, whatever the conditions. This is where I began to experiment with counting and matching my pace against my in and out breaths. To start with three out to one in worked unless it was windy and took my breath away, then I would have to increase the exhale breaths. I did actually learn over the next few weeks to adjust to different conditions quite well, the main trick being to learn to adjust your pace and breathing ratio to allow you to continue walking without having to have 'pit stops'. I was very relieved however, to once again get a car.

Also, pay attention to the length of your stride, this can make a difference to your breathing pattern. Don't try to take giant strides, aim for comfortable ones that don't cause as much exertion. You may find, when you're having a bad 'air' day that shortening your stride alone makes walking easier.

Try using pursed lip breathing for any activity. Breath out as you exert, whether lifting, pushing, pulling or whatever. You may also need to exhale harder as the

Who says I can't?

level of activity increases. When you are going up stairs, try different techniques to see what works for you. If your breathing isn't too bad you may be able to exhale up say two stairs and inhale up one. If you really struggle, try exhaling up one stair then inhaling without moving. Just climb one stair each time you exhale. You know when you get the ratio right as you find you can keep moving at the same pace, and it is so gratifying to have regained some control over your breathing! Try it! Do it now! How well you learn to do this is going to affect everything else you do for the rest of your life. Don't see it as a problem (negative), see it as a challenge (positive). Ask your family to help you and work with you. You will have taken a major step towards regaining some control over your destiny! The trick is to always stay mindful and in control of your breathing whenever you need to exert yourself.

Another observation which I am surely not alone in, but never seem to hear mentioned by any medical staff or patients, is a side effect of severe breathlessness. If I was silly (which of course, I'm not...usually), I could still run up a short flight of stairs even now, as my muscles work normally. The problem doesn't occur straight away. When I reach the top, there is a time delay before the muscles I have just used demand more oxygen. This is about seven seconds for me (consistently). As my lungs cannot possibly meet the new demand I would end up really struggling to breathe. Yes of course I should pace myself correctly, but as anyone with emphysema will tell you, "if I had a penny for every time I messed up with breathing I would be very rich by now!"

It's not the breathing that is the issue here, as I said, I have learnt to handle that. With extreme breathlessness, it's the sudden feeling that I am about to lose control of my bladder and bowels. They are wanting to empty and I have all on stopping them. It's only when I regain control of my breathing that this goes away. It is a very unpleasant feeling. It seems to be a reflex that happens to people near asphyxiation, as in hanging, so I guess it's just a reminder of how bad severe breathlessness is. This would happen if I got caught in a heavy downpour of rain and tried to 'hurry' (COPD hurry) to the nearest shelter. It is a bit personal and I have got away with it up to now, I just thought I should mention this in case anyone else has experienced it. If you have, slow down, you are tackling too much, too quickly. Is it just me that pushes boundaries? I don't think so.

Experimenting with, and mastering, pursed lip breathing, is one of the best things you can do to help stay active.

Breathlessness – Note for Health Professionals

A common, and very frustrating thing I have seen and experienced so many times over the years, is a well-intentioned health professional trying to restore 'normal' breathing in someone who is gasping for air. Yes, they

Who says I can't?

should be pursed lip breathing, and yes, you should be trying to get them to relax and return to abdominal breathing, and yes, they may or may not be 'panic' breathing...BUT...you have to understand that to go from distressed breathing to normal breathing is a **gradual transition and not simply a gear change**. There is a definite process that you have to go through from one form of breathing to the other. The times I have been absolutely gasping from overdoing it and clinging on for dear life to be told, "try to relax your shoulders and breathe through the nose". I can't! I am gasping, which means taking large gulps of air in through the mouth and out forcibly through the mouth. I have heard this said to many patients and seen the sheer frustration in their face. This is incorrect. You cannot just go from forced pursed lip breathing to abdominal breathing. Your body will force you to gasp.

Let me explain. Whenever you wish to go from an activity at one pace to an activity at another, there is a definite sequence of **changes to follow**. Imagine trying to stop a runaway horse by standing still and grabbing the reins, it won't work! You would first get up to the same speed as the horse, then grab the reins and only then start to slowly reduce the speed and gradually come to a halt. You need to go through definite phases. It is also the same process as if you are trying to break up a serious, heated argument. It's no good trying to step between two people arguing passionately by talking in a quiet, calm manner. No, what do you do? You enter at the pace of the argument and then when you are synchronised you can begin to deliberately slow the pace and calm things down. Subtle and deliberate.

It's the same when someone with emphysema is gasping for air. Join them at their own pace. **Talk at their breathing pace**. "Blow out, blow out, just focus on breathing out". Keep this going until you are talking at their breathing pace (which is being dictated by their body, not by you) for a minute or so. Now you have synchronised, tell them to slowly allow the out breath to start becoming just a little longer. Now a little longer each breath. Tell them to do this until they feel the 'panic' subsides and they feel back in control of their breathing (this is a very real physiological feeling as the gas exchange becomes under control again). Now tell them to begin to slow the breathing down very gradually and comfortably by continuing to extend the out breaths. When you see they are no longer distressed and start to breathe more easily and begin to relax then is the time to tell them to try to just allow the shoulders to start relaxing. When their breathing has really slowed down, then tell them when they are comfortable enough to start breathing through the nose to do so (if they can). Now tell them to allow the shoulders to relax each time they exhale. Continue to speak at the pace of their breathing. Now tell them to gently revert to abdominal breathing when they feel comfortable to do so. Now just allow them to compose themselves or sit in a chair or

Who says I can't?

whatever is good for them. WELL DONE, you have talked someone down!

Patients note – if you find yourself gasping for any reason and do not have your own technique then just follow the procedure above by talking yourself down internally. The key is to synchronise the pace of speech with the pace of breathing giving you mental control again.

As a footnote to breathing I have noticed over the years that if my work place becomes really stressful or is manic for a few days it really has a bad effect on my breathing. I know now to expect my breathing to deteriorate for about three days after a stressful period. You will probably have been advised to avoid stress but that isn't always possible, especially if you continue to work. I do at least recognise it and just allow it to return to normal gradually without adding my own mental stress.

If you find the subject of breathing more interesting than just necessary, you can explore it much more deeply if you join a Yoga or Tai Chi class. In Tai Chi (specifically Chi Gung exercises) we have many more subtle forms of breathing that produce different effects and are really fascinating, both to learn and to practice. We have Reverse Abdominal Breath, Scholar's Breath, Warrior's Breath and Bone Marrow Cleansing Breath to name a few. The spin off benefit of learning these is the strengthening of and control over, the breathing muscles. I have terrible lungs but have put many 'normal' people to shame when it comes to breathing! It's not always about what you've got but about what you can do with it. How well do you really breathe?

**Breathing is good for you...
you should try it!**

Oops...

A blonde lady wearing headphones enters a hairdressers and asks for a new hairdo. "Certainly", the hairdresser replies, "just pop the headphones off and I'll make a start." "Oh no, I couldn't do that", replies the blonde. "Well" said the hairdresser, "until you do, I won't be able to do anything with your hair". "Must I really?" asked the blonde looking agitated. "Yes please" said the hairdresser, quite firmly. "Well, if I really have to" the blonde reluctantly replied, starting to remove the headphones. As the blonde sat in the hairdresser's chair, she immediately began to gasp for air, clutching her throat and beckoning towards the headphones. The hairdresser, realising the blonde was struggling to breathe, didn't understand the connection but, nonetheless, passed the headphones to the blonde. As she was passing them she could hear the sound coming from the headphones..."Breathe in...breathe out...breathe in..."...oops, sorry blonde ladies. It's the only breathing joke I know!

Who says I can't?

Getting around – parking

If you ask me, even now, what is the most panicky thought that someone with emphysema has, it's what always goes through my mind whenever I have to go somewhere. "Will I be able to park? What if the car parks full and I have to walk? What if it rains? What if it's on a hill?". "What if" panic! It really does set all sorts of panic scenarios going in your head and is the single biggest cause of you failing to do something, because the thought of getting caught out is just too daunting. You or your family may already have applied for a Blue Badge (a disabled parking permit in the UK), which is useful to start with or on bad days, but actually has a down side as well.

There is no doubt that without the Blue Badge and disabled parking spaces there are a number of places I would not even consider visiting, like a town centre, but I believe that if you use the Blue Badge without thought, you are not doing yourself a favour as you will miss exercise opportunities. Maybe you struggle most days and need to use it, but just now and again you will have a good day, and those lungs need exercise, always be aware of this.

The trick is firstly to consider where you are going. If I go to the supermarket I have to consider a number of things. How is my breathing today? If it's quite good and the weather is okay, I will park near a trolley bay, so I get a gentle walk and fresh air, but still don't have to return

Joe Lodge

far with the trolley if it gets difficult. If it's really cold or raining I will choose a supermarket with a covered car park, so I can still get my walk. If my breathing is not good I will try to park as near as possible and definitely next to a trolley park. Every time you are going to use the Blue Badge think, "Do I really need to use it this time?"

One thing I have found is that over the years, as my lung function has deteriorated, whenever I park facing uphill, even on a gentle incline, my breathing is much more difficult, after even just a couple of minutes, because of the angle of my lungs. It doesn't matter if I am not staying in the car, but if I am for any reason, maybe just to get my breath back after walking, or waiting to collect someone, I always aim to park facing downhill, even in a car park with gentle inclines. I have measured the difference to be about 2-3% on my oxygen saturation (the difference between 'comfortable' and 'uncomfortable' breathing).

If you do have a disabled badge, use it wisely. If you can manage to park normally and walk, you will get the benefit, if not, you will lose the benefit. The way you should try to look at this is to tell yourself that **every time you do something that involves activity you add an extra day to your life, every time you avoid activity or someone does something for you, you lose a day**, it's a good incentive!

Also, if the front of your car seems to be a magnet (like mine), attracting all the buses and vans with smoking exhausts to drive just ahead of you, then don't forget that the fumes will enter the car through the ventilation system shortly after you see them. Close any windows, put the recycle feature on (if you have this) and try not to inhale too deeply. Wait until they have gone, then open the windows wide to clear any residue. "Grrr!"

Hospital

Unless you are lucky enough to have private healthcare, and like me, you rely on the NHS (UK) for your medical needs, you may find your first serious exacerbation leading to a stay in hospital, quite daunting. I cannot remember how many times I have been taken in by ambulance, struggling to breathe. When you are unable to manage yourself, it is actually a relief to be in hospital. After what may have been weeks of worsening breathing that I had assumed was just a bad patch, or work stress, I would end up, usually overnight unable to cope any more. I have often been frowned on for not seeking help sooner and I do try to react quickly these days, but having been brought up to be self-reliant, it isn't always easy.

When my breathing deteriorates I always pay attention to my other symptoms, is my phlegm green or discoloured, do I have a temperature? Quite often I would have no other symptoms, so I would assume that it may just be a bad patch and will clear in a few days. The pattern then would be to 'see how I am over the weekend'. If there's no improvement it's time for antibiotics. Unfortunately chest infections, especially Pneumonia can strike within days, so often, I would not reach Monday before I realised this was too much for me to handle at home.

During the period between 2011 and 2013 I seem to have been forever in and out of hospital. It almost became a standard routine. Usually late at night or in the early hours of the morning, I would ask my daughter to call an ambulance (these days she ignores my tough guy approach and calls them much earlier anyway). She would then pack my bag ready for the hospital stay. (Adding £20 for the taxi home while she 'borrowed' my bank cards!...that's my girl!). It actually became almost amusing, especially when the ambulance crews rolled up and remembered my name. Now I sound like a hypochondriac! It was really daunting at first, I was more worried about leaving my daughter on her own than about my hospital admission (Social Services please note, she was old enough to be left). It quickly became just a routine.

My experiences in hospital have mostly been good ones and I can't praise all the staff involved highly enough. We all know they are trying to give the best service possible, both because that is their job and because it is their caring nature that brought them to this profession, however, they do always seem to be short staffed and overstretched. I don't see this changing much in my lifetime as the advances in medicine mean more of

Who says I can't?

us are living longer, and often require more care from limited resources. So my point is this, if you have no experience of being hospitalised, remember that you are in hospital and they will help you recover. You are not in a hotel to be waited on hand and foot. You do not have an a la carte menu to peruse, and sometimes you may feel neglected. We all become a little selfish in hospital, feeling we are the worst case, well I can guarantee there will definitely be more patients in there in a far worse position than you, so have a little patience and don't moan and grumble if there's not quite enough meat on your plate, or you've been waiting an hour for another pillow. They will deal with your critical care, taking your observations at regular intervals, injections and medications are nearly always by the clock. It is a hospital, they will help you recover and send you home 'fixed.' What follows is my advice on how to make your stay most comfortable.

You have probably just left a controlled environment at home, where things are reasonably calm and orderly, where you have control over your meals and meal times, control over your sleeping, probably in a dark, quiet, room. You are probably now sharing a ward with maybe four or five other patients, so privacy is out of the window. Meals and mealtimes are pre-set. There will be new noises all night and lights going on and off, as patients groan or snore, as nurses come and go seeing to patients' needs. Culture shock!

As respiratory wards are usually populated by mostly elderly patients, they also often suffer with issues like some form of dementia (such as Alzheimer's), one of the signs of which is constant moaning or wailing, sometimes verbal abuse, which may keep everyone else awake all night. This, along with the constant coming and going of patients, nurses doing the rounds or waking you to check your 'sats' (oxygen saturation level) blood pressure and temperature means it is often like Piccadilly Circus at night. My advice, sleep as often as you can during the day and do not even worry about getting to sleep at night. Seriously, I have seen so many patients start to get stressed because someone or something is preventing them from sleeping, this in turn causing their breathing to suffer, creating more stress. Chill out! Get yourself ear plugs or better still ear muffs and a black eye mask!

The Golden Rule – when in hospital DO NOT expect to sleep at night!

To help you minimise your stress during a hospital stay, **here are a few things you need to mentally digest and accept:**

- My normal routine will now be different.

- I am unlikely to sleep well at night.

Who says I can't?

- Sometimes things will appear to run like clockwork, sometimes not.

- Sometimes I will feel well attended to, other times I may have to wait, especially if the staff are dealing with difficult or more urgent patient needs.

- This is a hospital, not a hotel, they will 'fix' me and I will recover.

- I will see many doctors, nurses and support workers, all with different personalities, some I will feel more comfortable with than others, but I recognise they are all trying to help me on my way.

- I will relax and go with the flow.

The Process

The hospital is an incredible 'machine'. Taking faulty patients in at one end and turning out 'fixed' patients at the other. You may have started your visit in A&E (Accident and Emergency) followed by Medical Admissions before a bed becomes available on a respiratory ward. This can be a daunting time as these departments are 'vibrant' (that was subtle) dealing with all manner of illness and injury, but things will all calm down once you are on a respiratory ward.

Doctors will have diagnosed your condition and recommended treatment, which will be carried out and monitored by nurses. At the same time, support workers will take care of all your needs and functions during your stay. Nurses then monitor and feedback your 'observations' to the doctors who will continue or change your treatment. At some point you will have recovered enough to pop out the other end. Sounds simple, and the physical side of your treatment really is straightforward. The area that can make your stay feel comfortable or not is the mental and emotional aspect.

Challenging wards

You may feel being on a ward with other patients a little overwhelming or intimidating, or perhaps there is a 'difficult' patient continually causing noise and disruption. As I mentioned previously, elderly patients with perhaps dementia or Alzheimer's are all too common on respiratory wards and it can be a difficult thing to deal with, especially when you are feeling ill and vulnerable. I have met this issue on many occasions. Particularly when they make continual noise, you may start with a polite "Will you please stop shouting?". This would soon be followed by a more stern "Enough now, please be quiet!", only to be followed by a more heated "For god's sake, shut up!" All the time you are getting more stressed. They almost certainly can't help it, so it is unlikely to change and may go on for days and nights on end.

There is sometimes an argument that 'difficult' patients shouldn't be allowed on the ward if they cause

Who says I can't?

distress to other patients but the reality is that the hospital have to treat them and maybe no-one could have predicted their behaviour, remember they too are in strange surroundings and may be just reacting as well. I have had a lot of experience of this situation and have developed and tested a few, simple things you can do to try to reduce your reaction to such things:

1. **Don't engage your mouth! (Is it just men?).**

    Your mouth is connected directly to your emotional response centre (inner child) in the brain, so as soon as you open it and make a request or comment, you are then waiting for a response. Of course, the response will be more of the same. While your adult brain may reason the situation, your inner child will just respond directly with more aggressive comments. Spiral? Yes! If you are easily agitated, try not saying anything at all to a difficult patient so you don't stir your inner child.

2. **Imagine a bubble surrounding your bed area.**

    This is your zone and everything in it is your business and your responsibility. Imagine everything outside the bubble is someone else's business and responsibility. You may observe what is happening outside your bubble but you now CAN CHOOSE to ignore it. You are safe in your bubble. This helps you to stay emotionally 'distant' and in control, much better for your stress levels, breathing and recovery. It sounds a bit too simple but I have found this very effective in situations where other patients are stressed and complaining. I have remained calm and relaxed.

With a little practice, you will find it easy to ignore a loud or difficult patient or situation, while at the same time allowing you to pay immediate attention to a person or situation SHOULD YOU CHOOSE TO. You are now in control, not your inner child.

3. **Don't do Patient Watch.**

    While there is always a certain level of patient self-management on a ward, unless you are calm and in control, don't mentally volunteer yourself for automatic patient watch. Sometimes the staff may be tied up with another patient and you notice the 'difficult' or wobbly patient is getting out of his or her chair possibly with an ensuing fall. "Nurse, he's getting out of his chair". "Nurse, he's getting up again". "Nurse, he's going to fall". "Nurse". "Nurse". "Nurse". You can easily get too involved and take mental responsibility for another patient, getting yourself worked up and stressed. If it bothers you, stop it. There will be other patients on watch, leave it to them and the staff, while you relax back into your bubble.

4. **Patients are people.**

    If you learn a little about a disruptive patient, maybe from staff or relatives you will find your

Who says I can't?

tolerance level will increase as you understand better that it is only a symptom of how they are and not the person themselves.

I am not by any means suggesting that any or every hospital stay will be like this, but I have found it a common issue that no one seems to be able to talk about or address, so I hope my few tips will make it easier for you, should you be in this same position. **Maybe one day I will be the disruptive patient next to you, if so, give me a wave and a smile to let me know my tips are working!**

Pain

In my experience, emphysema exacerbations cause more discomfort than pain. The pain tends to come from either injections or blood samples of which you are likely to encounter an abundance. The stinging pain of the stomach injection, given to prevent blood clots as you are inactive while bed ridden or the deep serious pain of the ABG sample. (Arterial Blood Gases). It doesn't sound bad but can be painful. "Just a sharp scratch" is the stock phrase. ABG is the hard one, as the nurse or doctor has to 'feel' about a bit to get into the artery. Am I telling you this to scare you? No, you may be very familiar with this procedure or be a virgin and have it all to come, either way, I am trying to pass on a tip. Pain (in this case) is just the body's way of signalling to the brain that there is a local intrusion into the body that would likely benefit from some attention. What is your normal reaction? To wince? To tense your arm or body? You are now focusing on that pain! The next time you are in this position (Oh yes, you will be, especially with the ABG's!) try to do the OPPOSITE. Try to mentally detach yourself from your body with the same attitude as though you were taking your car into a garage for repair, "Here's my body, do whatever you need to" and just allow the arm (leg or other area) to relax. Feel how warm and relaxed it is, what was the pain is just a faint hint of a message that will pass shortly. Try to make it positive, almost enjoyable and feel the difference. It doesn't come easily but with a bit of practice you won't care less when you see the nurse coming. I would say my pain level now during injections or samples never exceeds one out of ten no matter what is being done.

Deodorants and perfume

With emphysema I quickly learnt to avoid smoke and strong, bad smells, like bleach, hair spray and nail polish. Then it became obvious that any strong smells, good or bad, can really upset my breathing, so I would also avoid deodorants and strong perfume over the years, making me very sensitive if I do get exposed to them.

Now this is a respiratory ward, and I for one am struggling to breathe when I am ill, which is why I am in here. Strong smells, good or bad, not only upset my breathing, but I can taste them for hours. This is

Who says I can't?

extremely unpleasant and almost unbearable. I have experienced bank nurses with heavy perfume, families spraying deodorants, sometimes well-meaning staff who forget and give a patient a good dousing with deodorant after a shower. Sometimes even patients use spray deodorants ("why are you in here?!").

Nurses, support workers, visitors and patients, please, please, please! If you are in a RESPIRATORY WARD (there's a clue in the name!), DO NOT wear or use more than a faint deodorant or perfume. Thank-you.

Of course, being a man, the most popular and likely Xmas present I will get is...yes, you guessed it, deodorant! Doh!

Recovery

My usual reason for being in hospital is a chest infection, normally Pneumonia. If normal antibiotics are not proving effective, doctors would try intravenous antibiotics, which are a real sledgehammer and always work. Up to now, I will have been struggling with my breathing and feeling pretty ill, probably have lost my appetite and generally just want to sleep all the time.

Once the antibiotics start to take effect, there is a noticeable, physical change. My breathing doesn't feel quite so distressed, my appetite starts to improve and I actually feel like taking an interest in the world around me, maybe watching TV or reading a book. I know this is the turning point.

Normally, following this point, medication will continue and my observations (especially oxygen saturation) will eventually start to improve. In my case the staff are looking for 'sats' of between 88-92% initially and above this before considering sending me home to recover.

After the turning point I can just wait until I am well enough to walk again or come off oxygen, however, not being one to prolong my hospital stay any longer than necessary, I like to start my own process of Active Recovery (there's a new phrase?) a regime I use whenever I am in hospital.

While I would be the first to say don't try to rush recovery or push yourself, I believe from experience that my body recovers faster with gentle movement as soon as I am able to do anything. Of course, if I am advised or instructed by staff not to do something I will obey, I am not a rebel, just proactive!

I will probably have spent between three and seven days alternating between my bed and a chair, so I am not going to suddenly try hiking to the toilet. I would probably be a bit unsteady on my feet as the balance centre in my brain has had a little vacation and really needs waking up. I start my regime by simply standing up for a minute. This doesn't sound like much but there are a number of subtle things that happen. My heart and lungs begin to work just a little harder, so I allow my breathing to settle. My balance centre is now having to make continuous, minute adjustments to many muscles,

Who says I can't?

all the while monitoring my posture, to ensure I stay upright. Now I have its attention I will let it know I mean business by gently shifting my weight from one foot to the other for a minute. Then as I shift my weight off one foot I would also raise that heel so I am effectively rocking my weight on the balls of my feet. Now my balance centre is really paying attention, is up to speed and really getting in control of my balance, so I am ready to take those first, simple steps, with or without oxygen, it doesn't matter. I am now much less likely to be unsteady on my feet.

My favourite first goal is the window to see the outside world. What a tonic! It doesn't matter what the view is really, it's 'out there'. My balance will usually be fine by now and I will reward my efforts with a rest and maybe a biscuit before trying again. My ultimate goal is really the toilet, on my own and without oxygen (okay I know it's sad but this is what happens to my mental faculties when I am in hospital!)

Sounds silly? Too much detail? Over the years when teaching Tai Chi, I have observed a very noticeable difference in the students apparent balance ability depending on whether we have spent a few minutes stimulating the balance centre before we begin the actual movements, or not. The balance centre likes attention to detail. Also, I like to get moving as soon as possible because **external movement equals internal movement**. By encouraging my body to move again, I am gently massaging and flushing all my internal organs and stimulating my circulation, encouraging all my body's systems to return to normal functioning.

Medically, maybe my approach doesn't make any difference to my recovery time but the key point is that it feels like it does. When I was admitted, I mentally handed over control of my well-being to the hospital staff, now I can begin to take back some of that control and responsibility for my recovery. This helps me feel empowered in that I have an active input in my recovery time, which is usually very good. Who knows, I may even shave a day off my hospital stay ("shhh, don't tell the bed managers!")

If I was staff or a partner encouraging another patient in hospital to get moving, I would always make recovery fun, offering a bribe of a sweet or bun if they stood up or walked to the window. Our inner child likes to play, it does not like being told "you must do this if you want to get better." Tickle the inner child if you want to get someone moving.

Going Home

The hospital staff have done their job, as always, and my saturation level shows it is time to go. It may not feel like it, I always have to be wheeled in a chair to meet the taxi and when I arrive home it is always a daunting walk from the taxi to my door, but the danger is past and now the real recovery begins. It can take weeks, sometimes months, to fully recover from a chest infection,

Who says I can't?

particularly Pneumonia. I have noticed that as my lung function declines, recovery is taking longer, however I always do recover eventually. My biggest concern isn't whether or not I will recover, it is to what level I will recover. Each time I have had Pneumonia I have never recovered to the same level of lung function I had previously.

Anyway, you are back home, back to normal. If you have a partner or someone caring for you, enjoy being pampered for a few days, you have done well! If not, or like me, you have a job to return to, then a planned recovery is needed. Usually on leaving hospital you will have been offered a follow up by a COPD nurse and after recovery a revisit to a Pulmonary Rehabilitation class. Take these if you are offered, they will help you regain your strength. Medically, I would be advised to take a few weeks to recover properly, however, in my world that is not an option. One or two weeks would normally be enough for me to recover sufficiently to return to what is mostly a desk job.

I do not rush or push things but I do plan mini activities as soon as I feel able. I listen to how my body feels. If I can have a go on my treadmill on the slowest speed, fine, if not, just a potter around the house. If I can use my power ball to get my arms working, fine, if not, then maybe I will just try to wash the dishes. All movement is beneficial! All that matters is that I continue gentle, progressive movement.

After a stay in hospital, I always reflect on my lifestyle as well. Is there anything I could have done differently to prevent ending up in hospital? Is there anything I did in hospital that was really beneficial and maybe I should incorporate into my lifestyle? (Like not drinking as much alcohol...ouch? Got you there!). Sometimes a few small changes can add up to a big, overall difference. You are now home, take back the responsibility for maintaining your recovery and overall health.

Don't become a burden to your health provider, become a partner!

Ambulatory Oxygen

At some time after your diagnosis and pulmonary rehabilitation, when you should be at least managing your emphysema, your breathing level on exertion may indicate that you would benefit from ambulatory oxygen. This is available, after assessment, from the NHS on effective repeat prescription. I believe it is available in other countries but often at a cost. This is a portable cylinder carried on the back like a slim rucksack, that supplies oxygen via a demand valve called a conserver. This just allows a puff of oxygen through a nasal cannula each time you inhale. It's brilliant! It will enable you to tackle things that would normally be outside your scope. For me, it was the opportunity to do more hiking and

Who says I can't?

gym type exercises. It helps you to exercise and strengthen your body's muscles in a much more vigorous way than you would be able to otherwise, as it will help supply the extra oxygen the muscles need.

Initially, I had to be assessed by a progressively faster walking test, to see how quickly, and to what level, my oxygen saturation fell, and what quantity of oxygen was needed to counteract that. My prescription level was set at six litres per minute, which is the maximum available, indicating my lungs were not in very good shape at all. The nurse said it was unusual to be at this level. ("Yeah I really wanted to hear that!").

I was duly issued a number of bottles, which I could renew on a regular basis. Wow! Freedom! I was off into the country. If you are lucky enough (lucky to be able to have this facility that is, not lucky in that you need it in the first place!), there are a few lessons you will need to learn.

Firstly, depending on your set level, you need to plan your activity accordingly so you don't run out midway. At 6 litres per minute (6lpm) my bottle will only last about 2 hours. Of course, while I was instructed never to change the settings on my bottle, it quickly became apparent to me that I had to get smart as well, so when I stopped for a rest, which was very often, I would always take the oxygen off. A little thought made me realise that 6lpm was correct for rough ground or hills (full exertion), while 4lpm would cover undulating ground or paths (partial exertion) and 2lpm would be fine for level ground (light exertion) and this is easily adjusted on the conserver. This would really increase the duration of the oxygen. I did various checks of my saturation to ensure I wasn't causing any further issues (yes, of course I have a pulse oximeter which measures oxygen saturation, cheap and again from Amazon). Now, whilst the medical advice is absolutely correct and you should never change your prescription levels of medication or oxygen without discussion with your health provider first, I have found many things over the years that can dramatically improve my quality of life with a little 'tailoring'. Needless to say, my oxygen will last for a good 4-5 hour hike, or at least it did when I first started this years ago. Since then, my lung function has obviously deteriorated and I am no longer able to do long hikes.

The next issue I found when hiking is that I would like to carry a small flask, a bit of food and a cagoule in case of rain. You may be lucky enough to have a partner or friend to do all the carrying but I am an obstinate old boot and I have to be able to do this myself, if I can. I could easily carry these in a small rucksack...oops, I already have my oxygen on my back, so how do I carry a rucksack. Well, I was determined to find a solution to this, so off I went to my local hiking store. I found a rucksack just big enough to house my oxygen bottle in the centre, leaving room each side for my belongings. Solved! Or so I thought. When I came to try it out, it soon became apparent that the rucksack had become far too heavy for me to manage. This wasn't simply because of the

Who says I can't?

combined weight, but because the rucksack was designed to allow air circulation down the back, the effect of which is to hold the weight of the oxygen bottle away from the spine and my body's centre of gravity. This meant that it was effectively trying to pull me over backwards, requiring much more effort. So that was a good, new rucksack, confined to the ever increasing pile of objects in the cupboard under the stairs from my 'experiments'.

After trying various chest packs I finally settled on a very small, cheap, rucksack which I could put on back to front, effectively wearing it on my chest, with the effect of counter balancing the oxygen on my back, and keeping my posture balanced. I did find this was a real nuisance to get on and off though, so ended up with a good old fashioned haversack with a shoulder strap to wear to one side. I could have done this in the first place if I wasn't so keen on trying to balance everything, oh well, we live and learn!

I know of many people who have ambulatory oxygen but feel too embarrassed to use it in public due to looking like a diver with the added hiss each time you inhale, drawing attention to yourself.

I was like this to begin with. This is quite easily overcome and then soon forgotten, if you can just get through the first few weeks of being aware of children staring and adults glancing. They are just curious. Carry on as normal. You will probably find that your shoulders and back ache after wearing it for a while, this is quite normal and will ease once you make a regular habit of carrying it around, to the point where you can almost forget it is there.

One big tip with ambulatory oxygen. ALWAYS carry tissues, especially in cold weather. Your nose will run, the higher the oxygen level, the more your nose will run! You have been warned. If I go out with oxygen in winter, I would wear a scarf that can loosely cover the nose and cannula, which helps warm the air and reduce the runny nose. Even in summer, on the highest setting my nose runs and I need plenty of tissues. I believe it is just a normal bodily reaction to create extra mucus as the body has detected something foreign in the nasal passages.

Ambulatory oxygen is intended to help increase the level of exercise you can do, which it does very well. Another benefit, although unofficial, is that when I am having an exacerbation or recovering from a period in hospital, it helps me become mobile more quickly and aids recovery. As I recover, I just gradually reduce my dependence on it.

It is easy to start to rely on the oxygen even when you are not exercising, but a word of caution. If you regularly use oxygen, your body will get used to it and make necessary adjustments. Then, when you do not use the oxygen you will feel your breathing is very uncomfortable, so you will likely put it back on. This can become a self-defeating cycle. If, on the other hand, you go as long as possible without the oxygen (without causing major discomfort of course) your body will also adjust and

Who says I can't?

make the necessary changes to accommodate. After a few days you will find you are back to 'normal' and can manage much better on air alone, apart from strenuous exercise. This effect becomes more noticeable as your lung function decreases. Don't become an oxygen 'junkie'!

As mentioned before, I know a lot of patients who have been prescribed ambulatory oxygen but don't actually use it, as they feel too self-conscious in public for various reasons. If you are one of those and you would really like to use it but are nervous, try to find someone who already does, to accompany you a few times (Breathe Easy Group?). It is much more relaxing. If not, ask someone who is positive and gently sarcastic to accompany you and after a few outings you won't care what anyone thinks, or worry about the odd glance.

In the UK I think the NHS could improve the actual use of ambulatory oxygen if patients were offered an accompanied session for the first few outings, if they felt they needed it. I believe increased and effective use of ambulatory oxygen would reduce exacerbations and overall care costs. If the outing is with another patient, it only needs the health provider to coordinate it initially.

Self-Monitoring

Self-monitoring is a good thing when you get it right but it can also work against you if you are the sort of personality that becomes obsessive or paranoid. It is all too easy to fall into the trap of watching daily measurements go up and down and think that something bad is happening, when really it is only the body's constantly changing chemistry. Your temperature may be lower in the morning and increase during the day. Your blood pressure can vary throughout the day and one bad reading is just that, a bad reading. Ten minutes later you may get a perfectly normal reading. If you have a pulse oximeter and can check your oxygen saturation, this can be a really useful tool, but it is also the easiest to become paranoid over. Don't become a paranoid android, if you are this way inclined, self-monitoring is not for you.

In my experience, there are three different areas that benefit from self-monitoring:

1. **During an exacerbation** when your breathing becomes worse for more than a day and you think you may be starting with an infection. You may be lucky enough to have standby antibiotics, but still wouldn't want to start using them without being reasonably sure. Obviously, over time, you know your body and can often feel the difference between a bad 'air' day and a chest infection. You should always seek medical help as soon as possible in the latter case. You may be the sort that puts off seeking help for too long (like me) and in this case, at least some kind of monitoring is beneficial. Your breathlessness, phlegm colour and temperature are usually the best guide, although I have caught pneumonia on a few occasions and

Who says I can't?

the only clue was my breathlessness; then I would check my temperature daily at the same time (usually early morning) to see if this is rising as my body's first defence to try to fight off an infection. I may check my saturation but that only confirms what I already know, which is that my breathing is getting more difficult.

2. **During recovery** from a hospital stay or an exacerbation at home. You may have been 'pumped' with antibiotics, copious fluids and bed rest to overcome an exacerbation; often for me this has been pneumonia, especially in the early days. Whilst the pneumonia may be clearing, the road to recovery can be very difficult. I am always unsure, for a long period afterwards, whether I can recover to the same level of breathing I had previously, or whether my breathing has gone down another notch due to the permanent damage that pneumonia can cause. I have found that monitoring my saturation levels, especially first thing in the morning has given me clues to improvements before I have felt them. I remember, on waking, measuring my 'sats' at 92% for weeks, and thinking this is not going to change, it must be permanent, then one morning I measured 94%. Wow! My breathing didn't feel any better but that was a massive tonic! It was an indication that my breathing may be improving after all and was great for a mental shake up. Whilst my breathing may

have been improving, it was at such a slow rate it was hard to notice sometimes, whereas watching my saturation improving gradually over the weeks was a good visual indicator and a real morale booster.

3. **Regular check-up** – As I take responsibility for my overall well-being, I feel it is important to monitor my general health as well as my breathing. I do monthly blood pressure checks besides my daily temperature checks...but that is all. Again, if you have any doubts or are not confident to interpret measurements yourself, then have your checks done professionally and avoid self-monitoring.

If you do want to self-monitor and don't know where to start, the items I use are all available from Amazon or many local chemists:

Pulse Oximeter by Anapulse (around £20)

Omron M2 Automatic Blood Pressure Monitor (around £23)

Braun Thermoscan IRT4520 (around £68 now but newer versions around £40)

It was through self-monitoring I discovered many small but significant differences such as sitting back in a comfortable armchair leaves my saturation 2-3% worse than when sitting upright and is the difference between comfortable and uncomfortable breathing and this is

Who says I can't?

why, when I need an ambulance and they ask me to lie back on the bed, I insist on sitting up in the chair. When I am struggling to breathe 2-3% makes all the difference!

Just another note about self-monitoring; every time you are unwell it does NOT have to be because of your emphysema. You are still able to catch a cold or one of those viruses that 'goes around'. The more attention you pay to your body, especially when you have exacerbations, the more you will become sensitive to the differences.

If you do appear to have a chest infection seek advice and antibiotics as soon as possible. Maybe you already have standby antibiotics at home and have decided that you need to start them. Always remember, as your health provider will tell you, to complete the full course of antibiotics. If you stop taking them because you are starting to feel better, you run the risk of the few remaining bacteria, who are obviously more resistant to this antibiotic to have survived for longer, of becoming fully resistant and coming back to get you with a real vengeance!

Over the early years I could go weeks getting steadily worsening breathing, while arguing with myself whether it is just a virus that will clear itself. I usually ended up in hospital far later and with worse symptoms than I should have. I don't know whether it is statistically true or not, but it seems to be men who ignore symptoms for far too long.

IF IN DOUBT SEEK MEDICAL ADVICE!

Joe Lodge

One size doesn't fit all

If you are having trouble with a prescribed medication that seems to make you feel worse, after making sure you are taking it correctly and have given it a fair trial, don't be afraid to ask your medical carer to adjust the dosage or try a different medication. After an earlier heart failure diagnosis (due to emphysema), I found that the standard adult dose of water tablets left me completely dehydrated and feeling worse than without them. After realising that my bodyweight (BMI) is very low compared to the average adult, I reasoned that my dosage should be adjusted to match this. After agreeing this with my doctor, and reducing my dosage (two separate medications) we achieved the desired effect of reducing my swollen ankles (due to the heart failure) but without leaving my lungs completely dehydrated and solid with phlegm.

It is not wrong to question whether a medication can be made more suitable to your needs. Western medicine tends to take the 'sledgehammer' approach which is good during the initial stages of say, an exacerbation like Pneumonia, but when it comes to managing a problem over a longer period of time, the system doesn't cater for fine tuning of your medications unless you actively ask. As medications are designed to be most effective over the general range of average adult bodyweights, you may or may not fall into this category and like me, maybe find you are nearer to one of the extremes (mine is lower bodyweight). The usual course of action is to find the minimum effective dose, however that can take some time to become apparent, with a few adjustments needed.

Whilst doctors don't care for internet 'experts', there is enough information freely available these days for anyone of reasonable intelligence to thoroughly understand the dosage and potential side effects of their medication to a level that indicates a genuine case for suggesting an adjustment. Although my medications get reviewed from time to time, I do need to have an active interest in what I am taking, to what level it affects me and for how long I should continue taking it. After many months of gentle exercise and a heart friendly diet, I no longer have the swollen ankles and currently do not take any heart medications. This was my decision based on the premise that the heart is a muscle and therefore can be strengthened again to some degree.

Work

I am lucky in that I have been able to continue working throughout my emphysema years. I have always been an electronics engineer but fortunately, before I was diagnosed, I had been promoted to management, so no longer had to go 'on the road'. It's just as well, as this would now be impossible. I would struggle to carry a heavy tool box, never mind walk around customers' premises. My company have been good with me and never penalised me for my annual stays in hospital. They haven't really had to make any adjustments for me as my office is now on ground level and very near the car park. I was based upstairs previously and there was talk of a stair lift, but I would have resisted this for as long as possible because climbing that double flight of stairs daily was helping my lungs to exercise. It was also one of my daily markers, giving an indication of what level of breathing I would have that day.

As I work in a fast paced, commercial industry, which is often a stressful environment, I have had to learn a way of managing stress so that it doesn't overly affect my breathing. My tool for this has simply been Tai Chi. Any form of gentle daily exercise helps to ensure that you always return quickly to a relaxed place inside, no matter what is happening outside. If work affects my health at all, it is not usually stress that gets the better of me, rather it is fast paced action such as when the 'sh*t hits the fan' days and everything and everyone is manic. Phone calls, emails, actions, all become so fast paced I lose my breath and have to step back to calm myself and my breathing. The key to managing this is how quickly you recover. Thanks to my daily Tai Chi practice, I can usually recover from almost any panic or breathless episode very quickly and without any long term effects.

If you are still working, you are entitled to ask your employer (UK) for reasonable changes to be made to accommodate the effects of your emphysema (COPD). Maybe you could move to a ground floor location or have a stair lift installed. Maybe you need to adjust your working hours to allow you more time to get ready for

Who says I can't?

work in the morning or to shorten your day (with a pay adjustment of course). Maybe a small change in your job-role would reduce your daily stress and the effect on your breathing. Although your employer will be aware that they have a duty under Health and Safety regulations to consider your disability and make reasonable adjustments, I think if you are just open, honest and realistic about what adjustments would help, without quoting regulations, your employer will be more inclined to assist in a positive manner.

If you do not work, it is worth noting that having a daily routine that has to be followed is very good for your physical and mental well-being, as well as giving you a sense of purpose, of usefulness. If you don't have one and have the choice to get up or stay in bed, or maybe watch some TV, you will slowly edge towards becoming a stagnant pond! Everyone can create a routine. Maybe paid or voluntary work. Maybe helping those less fortunate like visiting hospice cancer patients or working in a charity shop. Even if your breathing and mobility is very poor you may be able to talk or listen to young or vulnerable people, which would be tremendously rewarding. Why? Apart from the obvious activity benefit, instead of feeing like you are no longer of any value to society you will cultivate a sense of purpose. You will feel that you have something genuine and needed to offer. After a while you will be motivated on bad days to still do your 'job' so you don't let someone down. This has the added benefit of your mindset becoming more concerned about others than wallowing in your own problems. This can help you remain so much more positive! Easy isn't it? Go on, think of something you could do to help others now! Imaging how rewarding that could be.

A funny little observation is that I am writing this so enthusiastically, I am making myself breathless! lol (oops, that's for texting).

Shopping

Even something as boring (for me) as shopping can be fun and beneficial. When it's cold, wet and windy, don't lock yourself away, go to the shopping mall. It is dry, warm, has lots of seating and cafes. You may be one of those people put off by the thought of too many people and lots of germs flying around, but don't be. Take sensible precautions. Make sure you eat and sleep well and feel reasonably strong so your immune system hasn't got too much to do. Avoid very crowded shops especially if people are coughing or spluttering. Don't touch many surfaces and if you do, carry a small bottle of antibacterial hand wash to use before you eat food. Avoid rubbing, picking or poking your nose, eyes and ears as much as possible, then stop worrying about germs and infections and go enjoy yourself.

I am not really into browsing shops at all, so I would probably head for a good bookshop to spend an hour or so and maybe try to park at the far end of the mall so I have a healthy walk on the way, instead of always trying

Who says I can't?

to find the parking space on the spot. I would aim to eat and drink just before setting off back so that I don't run out of steam on the way. With just a little planning I get some exercise and enjoy my day.

Never beat yourself up. If you find that you are having a bad 'air' day and just can't make it all the way, accept it and always have a plan B, maybe another shop nearer the entrance you chose, so that at least it's not a wasted visit. Always go with the flow so that you don't stress yourself and worsen your symptoms. As I mentioned previously, I have noticed over the years that if I have become stressed over something (not so much these days) my breathing can be affected for up to three days afterwards, so I very much go with the flow. Really, when you look back at the things that bother you now, in context most of them won't have been worth the worry.

Obviously, as I am a man, I may be missing a very vital point about shopping here and I would be the first to say that if you enjoy shopping for the sake of it, then go for it! All that exercise and excitement can't be a bad thing!

Another interesting angle on shopping is the supermarket. It may be that you are no longer involved in food shopping as your partner or family do it to save you the exertion. Maybe your supermarket now does home delivery to take the strain away. What? Stop!

The supermarket is a ready-made, all weather gym for you! Forget the weekly shop. Maybe even have the heavier items delivered to your home, but here is a chance to spend time walking in a comfortable space, away from the elements. If you can carry a basket, great, keep changing arms so both arms get exercise, if not, use a trolley. If I am feeling good I will put my ambulatory oxygen in the trolley without using it, so it's there if I get stuck. If I am feeling strong, I can wear it on my back, to improve my weight bearing exercise and reduce the chance of bone thinning through taking long term steroids and lack of weight carrying, common for COPD patients.

Carrying weights such as shopping bags, oxygen or watering can, stimulate the body's natural attempts to increase bone density, helping to reduce the onset of osteoporosis (brittle bones). Don't let someone else pick up the items from the shelves, sure, they may be light but you are moving and twisting your body constantly as you do this. How good is that? My supermarket has a pharmacy in the centre with a few chairs, good for a pit stop if I am struggling. Instead of doing a week's shopping I just buy a couple of meals, forcing myself to make about three trips a week. This is a good, gentle workout, especially in winter when I can't do much else.

Whilst I am talking about shops, a little rant to any smoker reading this book...SMOKERS PLEASE, PLEASE, PLEASE, DO NOT smoke outside the entrance to supermarkets, shopping centres and hospitals! You may be following the rules but you are making other people smoke, and I for one, just don't need it! You are forcing me to passive smoke. I dread walking towards an entrance to see smokers standing around it. No matter how well you think you are blowing your smoke away or

Who says I can't?

upwards like a chimney, simple physics will tell you that even if there is no wind, each time the entrance doors open a draught is created (because of the slight difference in air pressure and / or temperature, between indoors and outdoors) carrying your smoke towards the entrance and ME. I hate running this gauntlet, and what's even worse, is if I have to face it twice, once each way. The reality for me is that if I have managed to walk from the car to the entrance I will almost always need to stop to catch my breath. Likewise if I have walked around say, a supermarket, I will stop just before the entrance to catch my breath before attempting the walk back to the car. What happens? Every time the doors open YOUR smoke is drawn INTO the store and guess who has to breathe this in again? ME!!!!! I really want to shout at you and tell you how thoughtless you are. If this was happening to your mother/father/brother/sister you would complain too. DONT DO IT!! Walk well away from the entrance. Thank you.

Other medical issues

It may be the case that you have other medical issues besides emphysema. More mature patients tend to start accumulating various issues as the body ages, and of course, it's well known that as we have improved technology and testing, younger patients are now being diagnosed with a whole variety of issues that previously may not have been apparent until later in life.

Whatever you may have, don't deal with it as a helpless victim. Analyse how it affects you, are you making the best use of your medications? Is there something you can do better or differently that will make it easier to live with? If you are say overweight, instead of using the "I must lose weight to improve my medical outlook" approach, which is negative, boring and not sustainable, try " I want to lose weight, as I want see the look on my grand-kids' faces when I say I am going swimming with them!". Necessity is not the key. As mentioned earlier, my observation is that the medical profession tend to think that because you have a chronic illness or problem, you will diligently see the need to visit the gym and get fit. Wrong! People with chronic illnesses are still people, who can be tired, lazy, complacent, and generally want to visit the gym about as much as you do! Appeal to our passion! Keep it positive.

Stress and Emotions

Besides chest infections, another thing that can seriously affect your breathing is stress (and other emotions). Stress is your emotional response to events, situations or even thoughts. I already mentioned that from many experiences, if I have a really stressful day at work, it can 'wreck' my breathing for up to three days, not pleasant at all.

As your breathing deteriorates over the years you will notice more and more the effect of emotions on your breathing, say if you get angry or frustrated as a driver, or

Who says I can't?

maybe after an argument. Even good emotions can do this, for instance getting over excited. Think about how emotions affect your breathing now. Maybe not at all or maybe a tight chest. If they don't yet, they will. Think about the most common negative emotion you have and how that affects you, particularly your breathing. Any negative emotional effect is stress. Don't become a stress junkie.

There are two things you need to do, to get and keep this under control:

1. **Stop creating new stress**

    Pay attention to anything that affects your breathing and consider how you could change it. If you can't change it, can you change the way you feel about it? Does it really matter that much? Who is really causing the stress? How many times do you hear someone say about another person, "Oh they make me so angry". Do they really? They just do or say whatever it is, the anger is created by YOU in the way you choose to react. Think about why you react this way. Will it matter in a few years? Find a way to let go of the need to react. Try to remain grounded and not be tossed around like a cork on the waves. Yoga, Tai Chi and Meditation are all useful tools to help you remain grounded and more stress resistant.

    If you create your own mental stress by worrying about things or getting frustrated, it will not only affect your breathing but will accumulate and can then affect your immune system, maybe causing you to become run down, when you are more likely to catch a chest infection. If you have a bad 'air' day when you were looking forward to doing something, don't mentally beat yourself up about it, just accept it and do something easier.

2. **Recognise and dissolve old, accumulated stress.**

Review your stress life! Do you have bad relations with any family, friends or situations? These cause bad feelings and chronic stress. Think about what you could do to put them right, to stop the bad feelings. Settle any long standing disputes. Try to get your life in balance.

Try this experiment. Make sure you are in a quiet environment with no distractions, as this is a subtle experiment. When you are sitting quietly, comfortably and breathing normally, just pay attention for a few minutes to how your breathing feels without trying to influence it, just staying aware of it.

Now, one by one, think about ongoing things in your life (people or situations) that you feel may cause you stress and notice if just thinking about each one and how they make you feel, for say, a minute, alters your breathing, even a little. If they do, then they are a root cause of stress in your life. Make a note of them on paper to detach them from your

Who says I can't?

head and resolve to change something, no matter how little, about them. After you have finished making notes, list the changes you could make to the issues until you can think about them without any effect on your breathing. Although you should aim to make real changes, sometimes, just making the notes and recognising their effect on you may be enough to minimize or dissolve the effects.

Remember it is not the person or situation that is causing the feeling of stress but your emotional response to them. If there are major or obvious issues you need to deal with, then do this first. Each time you resolve an issue, do this experiment again until your breathing is no longer affected by anything you think about.

Congratulations! You are now a stress free zone. You will feel so much lighter in your spirits as well.

Comfortable emotions equal comfortable breathing!

Your Shrinking World

When you are first diagnosed with emphysema, you will probably have been less active for a while already, as your worsening breathing has started to affect what you can do. As time passes, you naturally learn avoidance techniques. "It's just a bit too cold for that trip to the shops today", "maybe we shouldn't visit the grand kids while they have colds", "I'll let you go to that show as the parking is really bad and there's an incline to walk up." It is much easier when you have bad 'air' days (or just don't feel like it) to find reasons not to do something, especially when the thought of the exertion or breathlessness is too much.

The natural reaction of a partner, friend etc., is to encourage you to at least try. This is okay sometimes. Just because you have emphysema, not everything is down to illness. You might be naturally lazy and just hiding behind the illness. You might just not want to do whatever it is. It is better to explain the truth, than always put it down to your emphysema, or allow others to assume it is, otherwise your partner or friends will start to build a subconscious resentment towards the illness, which will make them less inclined to suggest doing things in the future.

Listening to you moan about your breathing all the way through a show or during what could be a pleasant country walk does not pave the way to future outings. Better to be honest at the outset. Have a plan B that allows your partner and friends to carry on and enjoy the activity without you…AND without them feeling guilty about leaving you behind!

Your family and friends may also genuinely believe they are doing you a favour not asking you to go somewhere or do something, as they think they are

Who says I can't?

saving you the embarrassment of having to refuse or of struggling to breathe. Again just be honest, keep it light hearted with a sprinkle of sarcasm and everyone will be happy. Be careful that you think about each plan that you back out of, or you will find that offers of days out, visits to relatives etc., become less frequent. This is not a smart way forward, for you or your partner.

Partners

I have known quite a few COPD patients partners over the years and my observation is that they carry a heavy burden. Everyone knows what it's like to feel ill when others just don't appreciate how bad you feel. Well having COPD is straightforward. You struggle to breathe. You have days where you feel completely lifeless or ill for no particular reason. You have many reasons running round in your head why you shouldn't go there or do that. You can feel why. Your partner can't!

To start with they will probably feel very sympathetic and start doing extra things to help make life easier for you. They may have to start doing new things, jobs you used to do but find really difficult now. Everything will take longer than before. Just a visit to the shops can become a day out, as everything takes longer. They will do this cheerfully for months or even years. It is hard work being responsible for someone else's needs. Don't play on this! Do you remember what it was like to have young, demanding kids that left you exhausted, when you couldn't wait until they fell asleep so you just got that little bit of freedom, life, for yourself? That glass of wine started off as a treat but soon became a very necessary 'fix' to help you cope with the never ending exhaustion. Of course you loved them to bits but the reality is it was constantly, physically demanding. A partner with COPD is like that! A partner can easily end up quietly pleased that you didn't want to visit relatives or the shop, just to get some 'space' – not from you but from your illness.

You and your partner will probably both worry about leaving you on your own in case you have a problem, you won't! In all my years I can't recall any time where I couldn't have managed by myself if I had to, even if it was to call an ambulance.

The best advice I could ever give you regarding your partner is to make sure they have at least one time in a week where they are free of caring for you without feeling guilty.

It might be a night out with the girls or lads, a shopping afternoon, game of bowls or just time for themselves. What is really crucial is that it is genuine free time. It is natural that they will be concerned that you can manage and it is down to you to be completely open and honest to ensure they don't spend their free time fretting or constantly checking their phone. This confidence takes time to build.

Don't be a martyr! Saying "You go and enjoy yourself, I'm sure I'll find a way to cook a meal" isn't going to help, is it? We are all guilty of emotional blackmail sometimes. Poor me! Don't be so weak, you will be fine. Let your partner completely off the hook and they will come back relaxed, refreshed and willing to face another week's hard work. It will help you both cope. You will not feel so guilty that you are dragging their life down as well. This is really important for you both as individuals and for your relationship.

Try to keep your daily activities light hearted for you and your partner, a little shallow wit and sarcasm can get you through situations that may otherwise become unhelpfully deep. If you just can't go out now after all that getting ready, learn to laugh it off together. Maybe your partner could still go. Maybe you have a plan B. Talk openly and easily. If you allow the conversation to become too deep or serious it can start to create feelings and thoughts that might be too hurtful to mention or discuss, leading to introverted feelings of resentment. Keep it light!

If you or your partner find it difficult to open up honestly about how emphysema affects you and how this makes you feel, try finding an easier path like maybe writing a letter or email about your feelings. It is so important to be honest, then you can work together on new ways to handle life.

Cures

At this time there are no known cures for emphysema (or any form of COPD). I did however come across a diet (book) with supplements that allegedly reversed someone's emphysema over a seventeen month period.

Joe Lodge

Now any mention of a potential cure is like a candle flame to a moth if you have emphysema, so as it was described in great detail I decided that I would have to give it a trial. I hope the Trial Log notes (Appendix B at the end of the book) and diary extracts help to at least give you an insight into conducting your own trials with supplements should you wish to. The diet was based on the complete removal of sugar from the diet along with the addition of many supplements to help kill pathogens (virus, bacteria, fungus, cancer cells) and boost the immune system. I attempted to follow this as closely and methodically as possible.

The following are diary extracts during what I believe was a genuine and thorough trial conducted between 10th December 2012 and 26th Jan 2013.

> *Mon 24th Dec*
>
> *I think I am starting to settle into this routine.*
>
> *I have 9 of the supplements now.*
>
> *Medication – Acuhaler – I have not taken this for 7 days now which was my biggest concern, but if this stays ok it means for the first time in 12yrs I am not constantly pumping steroids into my lungs and subduing my immune system. My other concern is that the steroids reduced inflammation so I must ensure the supplements will make up for this.*
>
> *Still taking Salbutamol and Atrovent to keep airways max for the time being or until they*

Who says I can't?

become ineffective. Hopefully with the supplement boost to my immune system I will not need to take any more antibiotics (Co-Amoxiclav) and oral steroids (Prednisalone). For months I have been on a 2 week on 2 week off cycle as there always seemed to be a permanent infection lurking. If I am clear of interfering medication my body is able to restore normal function and I will add supplements to boost it.

As shopping has become a headache and to help with exercise, I have stopped the weekly shop and now go to the supermarket most evenings just to buy the following day's meals. This makes it mentally easier and is good regular exercise.

Prior to the trial I was doing exercise cycle/weights x 3 weekly + hiking at weekend (with supplemental oxygen).

Due to lack of carbs I have to subdue exercise for a while and tone down. Exercise cycle and weights gently with oxygen (to reduce heart strain) x 2 weekly...lots of small walks.

Tues 25th Dec (Xmas Day!)

Xmas day was difficult as I feel worse both in my breathing and energy. I think having no carbs, when I only weighed 8.5 stone to start is not the way forward for me. If I am to starve any pathogens of their sugar source surely they would die within two weeks of no sugar especially as I am taking supplements to strip their protein coating and to destroy them. I had a little mash and a Ryvita wholemeal cracker and felt better for it.

My new policy will be to revert to where I feel most benefit, so I am restarting my breakfast shake to incorporate porridge oats. I will have a little wholemeal bread with lunch and maybe potato with my tea until I feel strong again. If my breathing improves I will add to this.

As my emphysema occurred because of my Alpha 1 Antitrypsin deficiency I must be careful. If I restore and then boost my immune system I will also risk more damage from the deficiency. I understand someone with Alpha 1 may go their whole life without realising they have it, it would seem that if I had not smoked for 20yrs, I may never have developed emphysema. So the key is to avoid the infections in the first place. The supplements I am taking should boost my first line defence against pathogens entering my body. The anti-pathogen supplements should help destroy them if they get through.

It is 8 days without the Accuhaler now and I am sure this will be a good thing in the long run, however I think it is the main reason for my breathing, especially during exercise, to have

Who says I can't?

deteriorated. My 'sats' at rest are still around 96% and I can tease them up to 97/98% with gentle abdominal breathing. This will also help strengthen the diaphragm muscles which I have neglected lately. My 'sats' do return to normal quite quickly which is a good sign, as is my breathlessness, it used to be an awful feeling but now it's much more like normal breathlessness...only someone with emphysema could understand this, normally my lungs feel like a lead balloon when I am breathless but now they seem to be a little more flexible as though they have regained some elasticity. I know this is probably just subjective as it is very early days but it feels much better.

Wed 26th Dec

Time to review where I'm going. I feel very drained and always hungry. Breathing is still rubbish on exertion. I am waking up about six times during the night to urinate. I am dehydrated and need to drink constantly day and night. Although I think things are heading in the right direction it's time to adjust the method.

I have Googled 'side effects' to all the supplements and was surprised at what I found. Beta Glucan apparently can cause frequent urination so I am reducing this to 1 tablet per day. Apparently too much protein in the body causes dehydration so I am reducing the protein shake and reviewing my diet. Omega 3.6.9 can apparently cause inflammation, and as this is my greatest enemy I am reducing these to 2 per day. There is even a study done on mice that showed NAC (supplement) to cause PAH (Pulmonary Arterial Hypertension) where the blood pressure in the lung arteries is high causing the right ventricle of the heart to enlarge. This is already a possibility with emphysema and a cause of heart failure. However, this has not been tested on humans and may be species specific. Given that one of the main reasons I take NAC is that it can apparently boost the Alpha 1 Antitrypsin function which I am lacking in, I am continuing with 2 tablets per day.

Changes: New diet will include potatoes, porridge and wholemeal bread.

Sat 29th Dec

Well this is not good! Only Wed evening I walked round a number of shops and felt less breathless than ever and my lungs felt more elastic, the following day I couldn't breathe, now I appear to have a lung infection! I now have to act as I can't afford the permanent damage this could cause. I have stopped all supplements and started antibiotics (Co-Amoxiclav) in an attempt to 'sledgehammer' the infection without invoking my

Who says I can't?

body's resources. I have been eating a seriously healthy diet, had plenty of fresh air and exercise, and taken a whole number of supplements all meant to prevent something like this. What has happened? I have green phlegm. Is this an external pathogen, in which case how has it got past all these new defences? Is it a pathogen that was lurking and has now flourished again as I have started using porridge and potatoes again to allow me to have energy to get through the day? Is it inflammation or fungus brought about by the use of different supplements, some of the side effects listed were possible inflammation?

Unless I get worse I am not taking my steroid inhaler or tablets as I feel these have been instrumental in damping any possibility of my body's natural tendency to repair itself.

I have to go back to what works. I need to finish the antibiotics and then use the probiotics to correct the imbalance created. The only supplement that has actually made me feel any better (knowingly) is inhaling apple cider vinegar from boiling water. I am going to try this twice a day to see what happens. I will suspend the other supplements and only introduce them one at a time for say, two weeks to see if my breathing feels better or worse. I will use the standard dose and only increase it if I feel better, to see if it is more effective. I will stop using any supplement that makes my breathing feel worse. The proof of the pudding...

Tues 1st Jan 2013

Well it's the New Year and I have spent most of the holiday period feeling hungry, breathless or ill! Anyway, I guess when you embark on a journey into unknown territory there are going to be ups and downs, so I need to settle down now into a routine that is both effective (as far as I can judge) and sustainable (I have to have enough complex carbs to get the energy to continue work). I finished the antibiotics and the phlegm is clear now. As I couldn't understand why I had an infection or relapse, I decided to investigate the supplements again, not for side effects but inflammation. I have been taking Omega 3.6.9 three times daily as this is well documented to promote health, however, digging a bit deeper I find that whilst Omega 3 is necessary and is not produced by the body, so has to come from supplements, Omega 6 and 9 are not only available to be produced by the body but may actually cause or increase inflammation! Needless to say this combined supplement has now been removed from my list. Instead I believe that eating oily fish once a week will provide the correct level of Omega 3 in a more natural way (good job I like fish or it would have been another expensive supplement!).

Who says I can't?

As of today my breathing is slightly easier again, and I have eaten better allowing myself some porridge oats and a slice of granary bread. If I was able to stop work and had a partner looking after me, I think I would have been able to achieve almost zero sugar, but having to work, shop, clean etc, means I have to ensure that whilst I keep sugar to the lowest possible level I must maintain a usable daily amount of energy. Also, as everyone with emphysema knows, more calories are required just for the act of breathing due to the extra effort required by the diaphragm and intercostal muscles. As I am back at work tomorrow I need to get organised. I will alternate between scrambled eggs with wholemeal toast, and oats protein shake with half a banana for breakfast. Lunch will be a pre prepared romaine salad with either fish, meat or chicken. Tea will be either fish or meat, with a selection of steamed vegetables and either gravy or sauce. Some additional baby new potatoes on the plate but I will only eat if necessary (at least I have the choice then!).

I am going to keep exercise gentle for now (daily Tai Chi and as much walking as possible) to minimise the energy requirements. I will try to make no more changes for a month and then review whether I have achieved any noticeable and consistent improvements (whether just feeling better or any actual improvement in breathing upon exertion).

Sat 26th Jan

Well let's see where this ended...I have just been discharged from hospital after a week on four antibiotics for Community Acquired Pneumonia!!... where the hell did that sneak up from? Was it lurking already? Has my 'reduced' diet weakened my immune system and allowed it to flourish? Was it just bad luck?

Trial Conclusion

Whilst I tried to conduct the trial as carefully and thoroughly as possible from the instructions given, my experience of trying to apply the same techniques to myself leaves me feeling cautious (and £150 out of pocket from buying supplements!). I will continue to try new supplements or therapies to see if there is any real benefit for me but the sugar free diet with supplements was far too complicated and far too harsh and I will not be trying that again or any other trial to that level. I hope my notes give you some insight into whether trying supplements or trials is going to be for you. I do believe that with the current advances in medical science, one day a cure will be forthcoming, however, I would not expect that it will be within my lifetime, so I'd better get back to living well!

Who says I can't?

Where do we go from here?

By this stage you should have an understanding of your emphysema and the medications you have to control it. You should have found new routines and adjusted your lifestyle to manage it reasonably comfortably. This is the time when you should start to feel that you need to do something more, something over and above just managing. This is a good sign, it shows you are ready to take action to improve and enjoy your situation more.

I remember reaching this stage and wondering what I could do that would be manageable, new and interesting. I had previously enjoyed martial arts in the form of karate but there was no way I could perform that kind of harsh exercise now, it would be just too demanding. I then thought about more 'intellectual' martial arts like Tai Chi that were performed slowly and thoughtfully and wondered if I should give this a try.

I also remember my first class. I copied the movement the teacher was demonstrating and after trying it a few times found myself huffing and puffing as usual, but it wasn't too harsh so I stuck with it. I could at least actually do the movements. As time passed I became more efficient in my posture, using less muscle and wasting less energy so it was easier on my breathing. I also found what I consider to be the main benefit I have had from Tai Chi ever since. It really lifted my spirits! In the early days I thought this was because I felt empowered but now I know this is a real physiological effect. For the first time since being diagnosed and not being able to do things, here I was learning a new skill, which I was really taking to. It was a great feeling, I had found something I could do on a daily basis that would be both enjoyable and beneficial and mostly, I could do it for myself!

As the years rolled by and I eventually started teaching my own classes, I learnt that the 'lifting of spirits' is one of the most recognisable benefits that students, or more often their partners commented on. Performing Tai Chi, no matter how simple and basic the moves, always leaves me feeling a warm, comfortable glow, always reminding me of a 'Ready Brek' commercial on TV some years ago showing a boy with an orange glow around him.

Without wanting to sound like a salesman, I really can say that the one thing that has kept my spirits up and helped me get through so many bad episodes without becoming depressed or giving up, is my Tai Chi. Now it is no longer something I do, rather it is part of my daily life, in the way that I breathe, move, exercise, focus and relax. Do yourself a favour, try it! (See later section!) Or anything similar like Yoga, Chi Gung or Pilates. Any 'mindful' form of exercise will definitely benefit you in many ways.

Try to find a form of exercise that is interesting to you and then check how you would fit in to classes. If you are not using ambulatory oxygen for exercise yet, then you may be able to enjoy Yoga or Pilates, with some exercises performed on a mat. Personally, I have always found that anything involving mats and floors is out of my limits, I

Who says I can't?

just can't breathe adequately on the floor. It may be that the class is designed for more mature or less mobile students, in which case why not give it a try.

If you do use portable oxygen for exercise, you should try to find a class that you can just manage without it, such as Tai Chi or Chi Gung. Not using the oxygen, so long as this doesn't cause too much discomfort, will allow your body to adapt and also strengthen your breathing apparatus (lungs, muscles, diaphragm), instead of adapting to oxygen as a prop.

If you do use the portable oxygen in a class you need to check first with the instructor whether the constant 'hissing' of your oxygen will be disruptive to other students, especially in a very quiet, focused, class such as Chi Gung.

It may be that the class have no problem with you using the oxygen but if they do not use soft background music and you could hear a pin drop, you may feel too self-conscious. The trick is to discuss things and be daring enough to give them a try.

It is time to explore how you can do more than just manage your illness. There are support groups to join such as Breathe Easy, where you will find encouragement, activities and a chance to swap notes with fellow duffers.

"Who Dares, Wins" SAS Motto

Part 2 Summary

- Always use your inhalers as though you mean it!
- Markers rock! Listen to your body.
- Improve your strength and stamina.
- Become a black belt in breathing!
- Remember – every time you do something active, you add a day to your life, every time you avoid activity, you lose a day.
- Don't become a burden to your health provider, become a partner with them.
- Make sure your partner has a regular, guilt free break.
- Exercise MUST be fun!
- Who Dares, Wins!

Part 3
Enjoying life with Emphysema

Enjoy life again

Once you have got to grips with COPD and you have your medications and support plan in place, there will come a time when you ask yourself "What do I do now?" You may have spent time trying to build your strength and stamina or maybe you are not the type of character with the self-motivation to improve on your situation. You may need your partner's, family's or friends' support to help you figure out what to do next. Don't just leave it to chance though. You must understand, you have reached a critical period in your COPD time line and what you do or don't do next will affect both your quality of life and survival time. I have seen COPD sufferers over the years get their medication in order, go through the basic 'getting to grips with it' regime of Pulmonary Rehabilitation, daily routines and life changes, only to then go into 'coffin dodger' mode, losing interest in life, attempting less and generally sitting around watching TV or reading and being waited on with tea and sympathy, effectively just drifting slowly towards the end. Don't do that!

Understand this. The medical system (NHS or private) will be there in the early days of emphysema and again during exacerbations, if you need them, but they will not be taking care of your quality of life. **THAT IS DOWN TO YOU!** You have the means to improve your life at whatever level you are able to. I would guess that if you are self-motivated you will already be doing something along these lines.

You should physically and mentally take responsibility for your own future.

Find your passion

Now I don't know about you, but when someone suggests I should go to the gym to keep fit because I'm a duffer, rather than become excited I just tend to groan. Maybe thirty years ago when I was invincible! But not now. Sure, I joined a gym after Pulmonary Rehabilitation classes ended but that fizzled out over the following months because it is just exercise for the sake of it. If it was that good, all the doctors and nurses would be doing it. Ask yours, I bet I know what the answer will be, although it's probably disguised as 'being too busy'. If it isn't fun, it just isn't.

When you reach a point where you've tried the gym and you are either ready to move on or you have become bored, it's time to realise that the real way forward is to find PASSION! No, not that sort (more of that further on), passion for doing something because it stirs your emotions. Maybe there is a hobby or activity you used to do and felt really passionate about, that you could try again, probably modifying it to suit your current level of ability. Maybe it's time to discover new things.

Who says I can't?

Ask yourself what activities really stir your passion? It doesn't have to be grand like climbing in the Alps, it may be playing cricket with your little grandson in the garden or sketching village churches. It doesn't matter, **the fact that you are passionate about it means you are more likely to do it, enjoy it, and be bursting to do it again.** (Unlike said gym!)

The easiest way to find out what stirs your passion is to talk about hobbies and interests with someone else, you will both soon know if your passion is stirred, from your body language, rate of speech and breathlessness! Forget about how you will do something for now, just focus on what stirs your passion.

The trick then is to look closely at the activity and find a way to actually achieve some level of satisfaction in what you are doing while at the same time indirectly gaining the benefit of building your strength. Maybe it's just tending to your garden. Well, instead of using a hosepipe to water the flowers, use a watering can. Each time you fill it, do say, five lifts with one arm, then swap arms the next time. This will help strengthen the arm and shoulder muscles while you are just enjoying yourself. It will also give you more time to inspect the flowers more closely than maybe you did before. Really get into it, but keep looking for ways to build in exercise. This beats the gym any day! Maybe you used to enjoy horse riding but can't breathe with all the jolting now, so have resigned never to be able to do it again. Perhaps you could manage a led walk along a bridle path or maybe you

Joe Lodge

could help walk ponies with children on? Then you would have an activity to look forward to and get the benefits of fresh air and walking. Start by making a list of anything that stirs your passion, ready to discuss with someone. Go on, do it now! No really, stop and do it now!

Really try to spend time doing this, it can take you from talking with regret about everything you used to do but can't do now, to relating your latest adventure! How good would that be for you, your family and friends? It can put the spark back into your life as you realise there are still things you can do and levels you can achieve.

Through your initial days of getting to grips with emphysema, you may have taken up energy saving hobbies and interests like surfing the internet, reading and TV. Now is the time to think about this. Save those for bad 'air' days or winter. It's time to find activities with **MOVEMENT**. It doesn't have to be strenuous. Maybe learn to play the guitar or juggle. Maybe pot your own plants instead of buying them ready potted. What about learning to play a musical wind instrument or singing, how good is that for your lungs as well as being fun?! Find hobbies with easy movements, your body will love you and reward you for this. Your grand kids will love it!

Now you have to do everything much slower, you are blessed with the gift of time! Share it. While your family and friends are running around like headless chickens trying to pay the mortgage and bills and hardly have time for each other, sticking the kids in front of a computer or TV, you can give them this valuable gift, your unhurried

Who says I can't?

time. Get a magnifying glass and take a very slow, inch by inch tour of your garden with the grand kids, see how many insects you can find. You are really lucky to have discovered this precious gift, don't waste it!

Have you forgotten how to be spontaneous? When you next see a rainbow, stick the grand kids in the car and tell them you are off on an adventure to find the end of the rainbow. After some miles they will begin to realise that it just isn't that simple. Time to stop for cakes and ice cream while you explain all about refraction...you can, can't you? Wow, adventure and science! (You're going to look it up now, aren't you?).

Analyse and challenge the way you talk to yourself. Think about the difference between these two statements that you are likely to make internally. "Come on Joe, get off your backside, you really MUST do these exercises to maintain your health (or you're going to die sooner)". This is negative. "Come on Joe I can't wait, let's do some exercises now, it's going to be so much fun rowing that boat tomorrow!" This is positive. Which one can you get passionate about? Which do you think is likely to be more motivating? Think about this each time you begin to talk to yourself internally, or to your partner with COPD. Your subconscious will immediately pick up on this. Are you presenting a gloomy hurdle to be overcome (almost a threat) or a positive reward to be had? Get smart.

Even tasks that 'need' doing can be tackled if you try to look at them from a fresh angle incorporating something you have some passion for. I hate ironing but find it quite amusing when I either do it to music or Tai Chi movements (not sure if that's dangerous or maybe I should upload to You Tube and start a new trend?).

Think, speak and act positively, it really does make all the difference.

Micro Activity

In the early days of emphysema, you are mostly scared about exertion. "What if I put a strain on my heart?", "What if my lung collapses?" What you need to understand is that it's okay to be mindful about activities and not over strain yourself, but at the same time, the worst thing you can do is stop being active. For instance, my garden had become neglected. Over the years following diagnosis, I found the maintenance jobs just too much to tackle. Painting the fence was something I used to polish of in a few hours but as my emphysema progressed it became an enormous task and fell by the wayside. The borders became overrun with weeds, and again, this used to be a job that could be tackled with a rake, spade, bin bags and elbow grease, but after emphysema it became, "I don't like kneeling or bending, I can't breathe, anyway it would take forever. Yes, please do it for me". This mindset gradually allows you to excuse yourself from most activities and whilst you may

Who says I can't?

have family or friends support, who will rally round and get stuck in, sorting it in no time, it leaves two really important issues in its wake, physical and mental decline.

It's really good when family, friends and work support you by relieving you of the burden of so many 'impossible' tasks. They believe, quite rightly, this is the thing to do. However, **the less you do, the less you can do**. Your world of activity is in danger of a very gradual decline as you adopt the 'correct' response to offers of help, especially on bad days where everything is just too much effort. This is not good for your lungs or heart. Remember, your challenge is to keep them in the best shape possible, so **YOU NEED ACTIVITY**! Also remember, while all your focus tends to be around your breathing, it's not just your lungs you have to care for, you have the rest of your body as well, your joints, muscles, organs, all need movement to keep them in good order and full of fresh oxygen and nutrients. Imagine every time you are active you are helping your body become like a **bubbling spring**, full of vitality and life, every time you avoid activity you are allowing your body to become more like a **dark, stagnant, pond**. See the image, feel the image, smell the image. Which will you choose? The trick is to change your approach to the activity.

Over the years, you will have built an enormous mental library of tasks, washing the car, mowing the lawn, assembling flat pack furniture. In your memory you have stored roughly how long each task takes and how much you need to 'get stuck in' to get the job done. So when you view these tasks now and your brain compares what is required with what you have to give, there's no way you can tackle them. Wrong! It's time to get smart and review everything in a different way.

Almost any task or activity can be broken down into smaller and smaller chunks until it becomes manageable.

Read that statement again, slowly! It is so important! It is the key to doing almost anything!

It doesn't matter how much longer it may take, the important thing is that you can still do them.

You will have spent your lifetime up to now, doing most tasks without even thinking about what is involved. Prior to COPD you will have just got stuck in and done the task because your body (heart and lungs) was able to perform in this way. Now things are different, if you try to get stuck in to dig the garden or paint the fence you find within minutes this isn't going to happen. You collapse in a heap, give up and hope that someone will do it for you. Now analyse what has happened. You have tried to do something the old way. Not only couldn't you do this physically, but mentally you have just added another "thing I can't do" to your growing list. The mental list will eventually become "I can't do anything".

Obviously your heart and lungs will decline with less activity, but also think about what this does to your self-confidence. Remember when you stood back and admired the newly painted fence with your sense of satisfaction that you did this, your way and to your standards. You felt good about this when someone

Who says I can't?

commented on how well the fence looked. Can you remember these warm, ego stroking feelings? After COPD they begin to change. As you do less, you have less satisfaction about what you did yourself and more frustration about what you can't do now. I have known a number of emphysema patients and in private (usually because they don't want to upset their partners) they would tell me how frustrated they felt when they couldn't mow the lawn or wash the car any more, especially the men who were used to being relied on for all those jobs around the house, (male pride?). This feeling of frustration erodes the self-esteem and confidence and can easily become self-resentment and a negative part of your life. **DON'T LET THIS HAPPEN!**

"It is better to light one candle than to curse the darkness" Chinese proverb

On the following pages are my examples of Micro Activity to show you how I have used this technique to achieve many things I didn't think I would be able to.

Joe Lodge

Micro Gardening

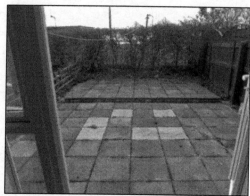

Back to my sorely neglected garden. Over the last few years I had just stopped bothering to try to do anything with it myself, the tasks were just too daunting. I was so frustrated, I had always done things myself. My family had offered for some time to come around one weekend and clear it all up for me. This was a really nice gesture for which I am grateful. However, it still left me feeling annoyed and frustrated that I couldn't do it myself. So I got to thinking. Okay, there is no way I can stand with a fork or rake and drag all those weeds out so that I can paint the fence, but suppose I could break the job down into small, manageable chunks that I could achieve when I felt strong enough. I decided to forget the big picture and just focus on the first foot of the border. What tools can I use to help me to do the job? How will I break and fold piles of brambles into bin bags?

I have to use my portable oxygen for almost all gardening activities. Kneeling down on a mat is okay so long as I don't keep leaning too far forwards and squash

Who says I can't?

my lungs, so I decided to reduce the weeds to a manageable size first so I wouldn't have to strain myself. Using a pair of cutters, I found that I could fairly easily just snip all the main weed stems at about six inch intervals, then just pick them up and put them easily in the bin bag. It took a while but as I stood up to take a breather, I could see that I had actually cleared just one foot of garden without all the huffing and puffing and strain. I was delighted! This isn't silly. Feeling delighted releases feel good chemicals in the brain and does wonders for your pride and satisfaction...a positive psychological result! So then onto the second foot and so on. Okay, what used to be done in a couple of hours was now tackled in odd hours spread over many days, but you know, I cleared all the borders, and the feeling was great. For the first time in years I had managed to start to tackle my garden, not by paying someone or relying on family or friends but **ALL BY MYSELF**.

Think about this, if you look carefully at most tasks and see them as a challenge, you can come up with some really clever ways to break them down into small chunks you can do yourself. Not only that but when you show your family and friends what you have managed to achieve they will feel so good for you. They are probably used to you grumbling about all the stuff you should be doing but can't and begrudgingly agreeing for them to do it for you, now here you are beaming with pride and satisfaction!

Bring it on! The fence took forever, I painted half a panel at a time over a couple of weeks, but now I glow when anyone comments "Your fence is looking good, who did that?" You know I can't wait to tell them. Can you see the change in mindset here? You can develop this to tackle all manner of things.

After I had cleared the borders around my patio, I even went on to add over half a ton of white chippings along them. Half a ton?! No way?! Yes way! One section at a time, I laid weed control cloth, piece by piece with a rest in between, until after a couple of weeks it was ready for chippings. A trip to my local gardening centre to buy 6 bags of 20kg chippings at a time. They are very helpful and would load the chippings into my boot.

At home I have a small, folding sack barrow. I would get this ready, then do some deep breathing to help my muscles get ready for the scary part and then on with the oxygen. Grabbing a bag and lifting it out of the boot and onto the sack barrow whilst blowing out hard did the trick (also I had been doing arm strengthening exercises prior to this to ensure I could actually lift a bag). Then a good rest as my body

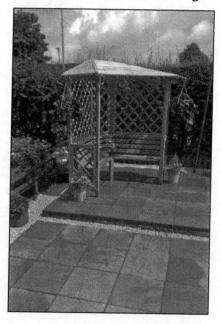

Who says I can't?

demanded oxygen to recover. Then push the barrow to my garden gate. Rest. Push the barrow to the area needed. Rest. Lift the bag off the barrow. Rest. Move the bag to the border ready to open. Rest. Slice the bag open in a way that would allow easy emptying onto the area needed. Rest. Lift one end of the bag and empty the chippings. Rest. Push the chippings by hand to fill the small area they would cover (normally people do this over a much larger area with a rake but that wasn't going to happen).

Finish smoothing the chippings into place. Rest. Take barrow and empty bag back towards gate and have a proper rest on a chair. Phew! Repeat. Yes, it took a number of days over a few weeks to eventually finish (remember I work full time as well), and when I did the maths about how many bags I had used and the overall weight, even I was amazed. Can you imagine though how good it felt? I am still proud of that task today!

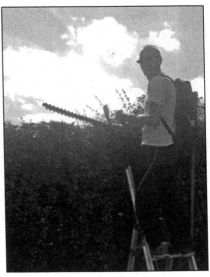

I even discovered that I was able to trim the hedge with electric hedge cutters, if I broke it down into ten second bursts with a good rest between. I would only manage about three feet on each burst but was I amazed at myself for doing something I thought was now out of my reach?!

"Gardening? Bring it on!"

Micro Country Walking

I have always had a passion for the outdoors, whether it is rock climbing, canoeing or simply sitting on a mountain or hilltop and watching the changing landscape. As my breathing has deteriorated over the years I found that not only could I do less but I had the added problem of negative anticipation, which is the hundred and one dreaded 'what ifs?' that ran through my mind whenever I planned to do something. One of the side effects of emphysema and the ensuing muscle wastage is lack of stamina. This for me results in going so far and then just running out of steam, sometimes I can hardly go another step. What if I run out of steam miles from a road? If I take my ambulatory oxygen, what will I do if it runs out before I get back to the car? What if there is an incline that is so hard on my breathing I just can't get up it or feel that I will cause my own heart attack? So many 'what ifs' become one of the most common mindsets leading to giving up on so many activities.

One summer, after I had built my strength and found a way to carry at least a cagoule, food and drink along with my oxygen, I realised I had to get smart about where I could walk. Using Ordnance Survey maps (large scale), I tried to find a route of say, a few kilometres, that

Who says I can't?

was circular, so that I could park my car in a strategic place near the centre and, if along the way I became too tired to carry on, I would know the shortest distance back to the car. It worked a couple of times but my local countryside (Derbyshire) doesn't lend itself to short, circular walks. This had now become a passionate challenge! I teamed up with a friend, realising that not only is walking alone inadvisable for someone with a disability, but if we both took our cars I could really get to work on the map. As it is always toward the later stages of a walk that I would run out of steam, I would meet my friend at the end point of the walk and leave their car there. I would then drive us both back to the start. See how this works? Leaving my car at the start we could set off with confidence. As the walk is no longer circular I could plan for two or three 'escape routes' along the way. This would just be finding a path that would take me down to a road, where my friend could pick me up, or ensuring that our route crossed a few minor roads along the way. If I ran out of steam, my friend could go on ahead and get their car (look, they did offer, okay!), coming back to collect me at the escape location. It was brilliant! It worked. I used it many times and it made map reading and route planning a real and enjoyable challenge. I couldn't wait to see where I could get too next! Of course, I never pretended to run out of steam just because I felt like having a lazy day sometimes, honest...

Joe Lodge

Whether you just like a gentle stroll or maybe painting or pho-tography, don't give up on the country, just get smart! There is so much fun you can have, even the planning becomes fun and the feeling of achievement when you get round a route, no matter how short, will be a great boost to your confidence, self-worth and give you something positive to talk about to your family and friends (besides lungs and breathlessness!). If you are useless with maps, see if you can get your family or friends to help, a short country walk can turn into quite an interesting adventure! **DO IT!**

It doesn't matter how far you walk, what is important is how much you enjoy it. If you spend the whole time huffing and puffing then you will remember it as a bad experience and be more likely to avoid it. If, on the other hand, you don't get far but manage to recognise all the tree names along the way as well as spotting that rabbit and capturing the most amazing photo of a cloud formation that looks like the British Isles, you will be as excited as a young child at the next opportunity to get outdoors! Your ability to walk further will then take care of itself over time.

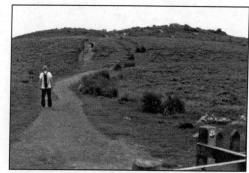

Higger Tor

Who says I can't?

Sometimes, even a psychological cheat is just as good. I like nothing more than to be on top of a hill or mountain, with the sense of freedom that brings, however, it is very difficult to achieve these days. There is though, a local hill in Derbyshire called Higger Tor and I used to climb this from the bottom as part of a long hike. There is a road running over the shoulder of the hill and now I just park my car a few hundred yards from the top.

It is still an uphill struggle and some-times can take me an hour with lots of short 'pit stops', but once I am on the top, it doesn't matter one bit that I have walked only the last stage. I am on top of my Everest! (I consider this upper car park is just my Everest Summit Camp!). The view and the surroundings are breath taking and I am happy to simply sit for hours taking it all in. I can return home completely recharged from this little adventure.

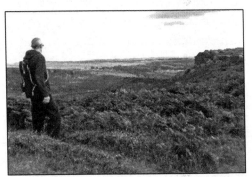

"My Everest"

A reminder: If you decide to walk outside, with or without ambulatory oxygen, in the colder months, make sure you have a scarf or something similar covering your mouth and nose...and those tissues!

Joe Lodge

Breaking a country walk down into components you can plan and manage easily makes it both possible, enjoyable and under your control.

Micro Gym

If you do decide to go to the gym, micro activity works down there too! If you are actively trying to build your strength for a particular goal, don't be put off by the wrong concept. Although I would not go to the gym just because I 'should', when I am working towards a goal, I do need strengthening exercises. As I find going to the gym very difficult anyway simply due to a busy lifestyle, I have bought the gym to me, with my treadmill, cycle and weights. Don't expect to suddenly be able to do thirty press ups if you haven't used your arm muscles for years, you will just see it as too hard and give up before you get started. Let me give you an example:

I needed to be able to lift my bodyweight with my arms to achieve a summer challenge, so I bought one of those bars that fits into a door frame so that I could do 'chin ups' (eventually!) This is where you lift your body weight with your arms until your chin touches the bar. Needless to say I couldn't even get off the floor! My plan was to micro exercise and break it into small steps.

- Just hold the bar and practice taking my weight without my feet even leaving the floor. Do this daily in three groups of seven lifts, holding each lift for seven seconds. Do this for the first week.

Who says I can't?

- Then repeat the same pattern but this time raising my body weight onto my toes.

- Same again but now just lifting my feet off the floor.

- Now the same but lifting towards the bar.

- Now touching the bar with my chin.

Sorted! It took me a little time, but breaking it into steps gave my body time to adapt and strengthen. You will be amazed what you can achieve this way!

I can currently do five chin up's anytime (without oxygen) which gave me the extra arm strength I was trying to achieve, and as a bonus, I get to put a lot of healthy visitors to shame!

Micro Sports & hobbies

If you have decided you want to try new things but don't know where to start, I would suggest making a list of all the sports and hobbies that come to mind. The internet is a great source of information, there may be things you never dreamed of trying that you might really take to. I started with an alphabetical list, but then I grouped them according to the level of exertion required, so water skiing would be near the top, while playing the guitar or chess would be further down. I will always try a new activity at the highest level of comfortable exertion I can reach at the time, by breaking it into manageable chunks if possible, the theory being that as my breathing deteriorates over the years, my enthusiasm for activity and learning new things won't. I will simply adjust what I am doing or learning to my current level of strength, stamina and breathing. Sometimes I don't get it right, I remember trying go-karting. Oh boy! A great thrill but three minutes of body numbing vibration later and I couldn't breathe! Oh well, tried it, done it, moved on.

Micro Canoeing

My desire for the last few years has been to go canoeing again. In my fit days I loved water sports, especially water skiing but a realistic option now is canoeing. A few years ago I found myself standing on a jetty at our nearby water sports park constantly wishing I could just get out on that water again. The sports centre hire canoes out but these are 'sit on – fall off' type which may be fun but not what I am needing or looking for. It is also mandatory to wear a wet suit which they also supply. Everything then is done against a time limit, not my 'best friend' and for someone who struggles just to don everyday clothes, getting into or out of a wetsuit would be really difficult and waste so much energy. Also, the fibreglass canoes are so heavy to manoeuvre when they tip over or when out of the water. Then there is the question of what happens if I capsize? Will I be able to breathe enough to swim to safety? What about the cold water? I can't carry my oxygen so it can't be done! Out of the question! Or is it?

Who says I can't?

Following on from my success in micro managing my garden, I decided to see if I could find a realistic solution that could get me on the water. Firstly, I accepted that there was no way I could physically cope with the hire option, I would have to have my own things, so I wasn't under any time constraint. As friends and family are always so busy, I decided I would have to be able to tackle this alone. I discovered that there are some really good and credible inflatable canoes on the market, but always more questions, how would I inflate it? How would I carry it to the water? (even inflatables are heavy for me). After a year of planning and wishing I finally took the plunge (oops...).

After listening to my constant ramblings, my daughter actually bought me an inflatable canoe for Xmas (No, she did not receive excessive pocket money, she was doing some part time work!). This was it. Time for action as soon as the spring sunshine allowed. It was quite nerve racking really. I started by finding a jetty which was the only place I thought I would be able to get in and out of the canoe without the traditional 'get your legs wet' approach. I had found a parking space for the car which nearly backed onto the jetty so I had minimum carrying distance. I placed a ground sheet on the gravel floor behind the car so I could easily sit on the floor to make it easier to tackle the tough task of inflating the canoe.

Now inflatables come with a built in pressure monitor so you can tell when it is inflated correctly. As it retains the highest pressure measurement, this is what the manufacturer will use if you return your canoe as faulty under warranty, to determine if you have over inflated it. The instruction manual states clearly DO NOT use an electric pump for this reason, use a foot pump. Likely!

This was my first big hurdle. My solution was to ignore the manufacturers warning and accept that if I split the seams it would be my own stupid fault. Using an electric pump carefully would get the canoe 90% inflated and I could just 'tweak' it then with the foot bellows (and oxygen!). This was still the hardest and longest part of preparation. Pump, pump, rest, pump, pump, rest...

After resting I would strap on my oxygen and carry the canoe to the edge of the jetty. This wasn't actually as hard as I expected. Again I would rest. In with the seats and paddle. Rest. On with my life jacket and whistle. Rest. I had tried to create a flotation device for my oxygen bottle but realised it could never work as the air tube had to come through a hole, so I broke the rules (again, oops) and wedged and tethered the bottle into the back part of the canoe behind my seat. I figured that as the canoe has separate sections for inflation, even if I had a puncture in one and ended up in the water, there would still be enough flotation for my oxygen. I could then tread water until help came. I do have a whistle and there is a safety boat patrolling. How will I be able to blow a whistle if I am struggling to breathe? Easy...don't panic, take my time until my breathing is under control. Risky? Stupid? Yes, some people thought I was irresponsible, but I grew up in the days where boys could play conkers without wearing safety goggles and gloves. Getting hurt was part

Who says I can't?

of the learning curve. If I don't take some calculated risks sometimes, I will never have fun!

So, I had the canoe on the jetty all ready to go. I then slid it into the water and tethered it to the railings around the jetty so I could return to the car for a small snack and drink before I set off. Getting into the canoe left me breathless, because it meant taking my weight onto my arms while attempting a quick bum slide off the jetty into the centre of the canoe, and all without tipping over! Actually, inflatable canoes are almost unsinkable, I think I should call mine 'Titanic'...okay, maybe that's pushing it? I think I probably looked a bit silly..."Mum look at that old man over there in that toy boat, it's taken him hours to get in the water". Hey, I long since stopped caring what people think, I will soon be paddling to my heart's content on the water I love so much, while they just sit on their backsides eating ice cream before going home to slouch in front of the TV.

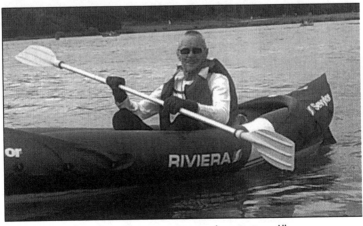

"Eat your heart out, couch potatoes!"

Okay, it took me about two hours to get on the water and after thirty minutes paddling I was exhausted, but I DID IT! Another hour to pack away. So my "Done anything this weekend?" response had changed from "Well, I managed to walk round the supermarket but my breathing's not so good" to "Yeah, I went canoeing" **"What?! No way?! Yes way!"**

I hope the examples of micro activity above demonstrate that almost anything can be tackled if you break it into small steps, pay attention to detail and see it as a fun challenge. Don't focus on the big picture, just on the next step and you will eventually arrive at your goal. Stop for a moment now and think about something you would really like to do? How could you break it into small steps and actually enjoy it?

Imagine how tickled your loved ones would be to see you with a smile and a glint in your eyes, when they ask "What on earth are you up to now?"

I can almost hear those chuckles and see those smiles as you have little eureka moments when you discover how to do something you thought was out of your grasp! "Yes!"

REMEMBER – Everything you do for yourself adds to your lifespan, everything you avoid or someone does for you, subtracts from your lifespan...try to do everything yourself, just in a different way!

Who says I can't?

Smart targets

Smart targets are a great way of ensuring that when you plan something, it is achievable. It is not rocket science but a simple way of just checking you have thought your plans through, so you can actually achieve a measurable target, even a small one. There is much information about this on the internet so I will only mention the basic outline. I use SMART targets to check that the challenges I set for myself are realistic. There's nothing like a challenge to get the adrenaline pumping!

SMART stands for:

Specific – make sure you set a specific target. Don't say this week I want to walk a lot more, say this week I want to walk 1km more than last time.

Measurable – make sure you will be able to compare what you plan to achieve against what you actually achieve, using distance, time, weight or whatever is applicable.

Achievable – make sure it is actually possible within your limits. Don't set a target of a 10kms walk if you have only ever done 3kms. Try to go for 4 or 5.

Realistic – the target should be at level you are willing, able and enthusiastic enough to try achieving.

> **Timely** – give yourself a specific deadline. This week or within six weeks. This is easier and more motivating than an open ended time scale.

Whenever you make plans, just run them past SMART to make sure they will bring you the satisfaction of saying "I did that myself!"

Example – my 2015 Challenge...climb the Flying Buttress on Stanage Edge near Sheffield.

> **Specific** – climb the classic HVD (hard very difficult, classification) route up the left side of the Flying buttress with a top rope for safety.
>
> **Measurable** – simple...if I get to the top, no matter how long it takes, I have climbed it!
>
> **Achievable** – I can climb two sets of stairs at work with rests on the way, if I can increase my strength and stamina over the next few months, and I use very careful and deliberate movements, I believe I can do this.
>
> **Realistic** – last year I managed canoeing after a year of wishing and planning, I need my target to stretch my limits. I know I can rest at the top of the first section before the crux (hardest part) of the climb, so this can be done...so long as my oxygen bottle doesn't make climbing too difficult! ...I will watch other climbers many times to know exactly how to place my hands and feet so I don't waste energy.

Who says I can't?

Timely – I must do this during the summer months while the rock is warmer.

Note – there is no such thing as failure. The only way to fail at something is never to attempt it! If I don't succeed on the first attempt, (whether it's climbing rocks or painting the fence) I will analyse why and learn from it by adapting my approach. If I still don't succeed I will change the climbing route to avoid or overcome the problem until I do achieve success.

"Improvise, adapt and overcome" – **US Marines Motto** and three very powerful words when you apply them to any challenge in life.

Why do it? – Because it's there! I am going to spend many hours on the treadmill and using weights to get ready for this challenge. This is fun. I am not getting fit just because I'm supposed to.

I will need to visit the area many times before the climb, and as the access to Stanage Edge is via a fairly steep (to me) uphill path, I will get the added benefit of exercise and fresh air, all with a sense of purpose.

I will be so much stronger and healthier to go into the winter months, which has to be good for my immune system. Mostly though, I just can't turn down a challenge! (Even though it's my own).

Joe Lodge

Tai Chi Taster (Micro Tai Chi !)

Now for something much slower. As I have such passion for Tai Chi, I cannot let you escape without inviting you to at least try a little taster session. It will only take about fifteen minutes of your time and it doesn't matter whether you are a patient, partner, family, friend or carer, just have a go for fun. If you don't have time right now, then come back to this when you do. It is not just a couple of moves for you to try but an example of a real 'warm up' session I would use at the beginning of a class.

If you follow the instructions until you can repeat the simple movements in a slow and deliberate manner, you should find that it leaves you feeling pleasantly relaxed. Even this simple routine, repeated daily, will help improve your sense of well-being and self-help. If you do enjoy it and decide to attend a class, then good for you. If not, at least you will have a little routine you can use to get you 'moving' in a relaxed way.

I have written it so that it can be read as a script, as you can't be reading the instructions at the same time as following them, so if you can't memorise the instructions (in chunks), you can ask someone to read the instructions to you, very slowly, as you follow them or even read them yourself and record them so you can play them back. You could just learn one small section at a time, then add the next section. Don't think about analysing what you are doing or why, just relax and enjoy a few moments of mindfulness. These are very simple

Who says I can't?

movements, but if at any time you feel uncomfortable in any way, then just stop.

Whether you are reading this out for someone or recording it for yourself, it is most important to follow the pauses carefully, to allow time for the practitioner to experience and enjoy each of the movements before moving on, so read in a soothing voice, VERY SLOWLY and PAUSE or WAIT and do nothing, when told. You can make the mistake of reading this too quickly, but not of reading too slowly.

As you read the instructions, where you see a comma, pause for a second, where you see PAUSE, wait a few seconds...where you see WAIT, then wait for about 10 seconds and do nothing, to allow the person time to experience the movement or feeling.

Read through the instructions first and see the accompanying photos which should serve as a guide to doing the simple movements correctly.

As you follow the instructions, they may appear to be long winded, but the apparent time is distorted by me writing this in very fine detail.

Just ensure you are in a comfortable space with no distractions. Wear flat shoes or bare feet. Loosen any tight clothing and remove any tight or heavy jewellery. Gently shake your arms and legs before you begin. Try to just ignore any thoughts that pop into your head and just focus on the instructions.

Joe Lodge

Begin

- Now, I want you to stand comfortably with your feet about shoulder width apart and parallel (not toed in or out). PAUSE.

- Stand tall, but relaxed. PAUSE.

- Relax your knee joints a little so they are not locked. PAUSE.

- Just try to keep a comfortable posture, with the back and head straight but relaxed. PAUSE.

- Now allow the shoulders to relax and sink and just allow the arms to hang by your sides

- (Fig a). PAUSE.

Keep the fingers and thumbs open but relaxed and without tension, just as you would if you were holding a large ball (Fig b). PAUSE.

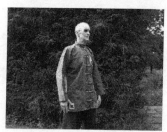

Fig a

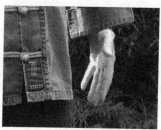

Fig b

Who says I can't?

- If you can close your eyes without losing your balance then do so. If not, just keep a soft focus to the front. Just experience this position for a few moments. WAIT.

- Now, pay attention to your feet, and notice how you feel your weight is distributed. PAUSE.

- Is your body making continual, minute adjustments to keep you balanced? PAUSE.

- Just observe this subtle movement. WAIT.

- Now, allow your attention to wander down your body, from your head to your feet, just allowing each part to relax as you do, relax your head PAUSE, the face and jaw PAUSE, relax the neck and shoulders PAUSE, relax your back PAUSE, your hips PAUSE, knees PAUSE, and ankles, PAUSE.

- Now, paying attention to your feet, just try to rock forwards very, very slightly, slowly and gently, to just move your weight towards the balls of your feet and hold it there for a moment. PAUSE.

- Now, allow your weight to just rock back carefully towards the heels. PAUSE.

- Now forwards again. PAUSE. Just keep doing this very slowly and gently for a few moments, keeping your attention on your feet and still keeping your eyes closed, unless you feel unsteady. Just enjoy this subtle movement, very slowly. WAIT.

- Now, just allow your weight to settle in the centre between the balls of the feet and the heels. PAUSE.

- Now, a similar movement, but this time moving your weight slightly to the left, gently placing more weight over the left foot and less over the right, slowly and deliberately. PAUSE.

- Now move your weight back to the centre, PAUSE, then to the right. PAUSE.

- Repeat carefully and very slowly for a few moments, centre, left, centre, right. WAIT.

- Now, just allow your weight to rest in the centre. PAUSE.

- Just relax in this position, arms hanging loosely at your side, PAUSE. If any part of you feels uncomfortable, just adjust your position slightly until you can relax and pay attention to the next step. WAIT.

- Now, I want you to shift your attention to your breathing. PAUSE.

- Don't try to control it, just notice it. PAUSE.

- Notice how long you are inhaling for. PAUSE.

Who says I can't?

- Notice how long you are exhaling for. PAUSE.

- Notice the pause between inhaling and exhaling. PAUSE.

- Notice the pause between exhaling and inhaling. PAUSE.

- Pay attention to these pauses without trying to control your breathing in any way. WAIT.

- Now, begin to inhale very gently through the nose and exhale very gently through the mouth. PAUSE.

- If you find this is difficult, just breathe through the mouth for now. PAUSE.

- Pay attention to your stomach, and allow it to expand as you inhale and relax as you exhale. PAUSE.

- Don't force your breathing, just keep it natural and relaxed. In through the nose, PAUSE, out through the mouth. PAUSE.

- This is abdominal breathing as described earlier. PAUSE.

- Just allow your breathing to settle. Usually after a short time you should notice your breathing becomes much deeper and more relaxed. PAUSE. Just enjoy this feeling. WAIT.

- Now, allowing your breathing to stay soft and relaxed, inhale as though you were inhaling a long, silk, handkerchief through your nostrils, softly, slowly, continuously, PAUSE.

- Then exhale through gently pursed lips as though you were trying to just bend a candle flame without blowing it out. PAUSE.

- Repeat this until you find it comfortable. WAIT.

- Now, each time you exhale, just allow your shoulders to relax. PAUSE.

- See how good this feels. WAIT.

- Now, each time you exhale and relax your shoulders just count down, beginning at 9 and counting down with each breath until you reach 0 and then just breathe normally and stay relaxed. WAIT (for 9 long, comfortable breaths).

- You should now be relaxed and breathing normally. PAUSE.

- Now we are going to try an arm movement. PAUSE.

- Just allow your arms to move slowly around towards the front of your body. PAUSE.

- Imagine there is a large, heavy, object in front of you. PAUSE.

Who says I can't?

- Place your palms flat on the heavy object, about chest height (Fig c). PAUSE.

- Now push the object very slowly away from you, keeping the palms on the object. PAUSE.

- Push it right out until your arms are extended. (Fig d) You should feel a little strain in your wrists, elbows and shoulders. PAUSE.

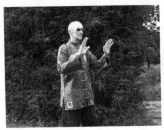 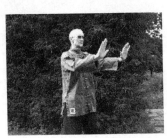

Fig c   Fig d

- Now just relax your arms and bring them slowly back towards your chest, allowing your elbows to just bend and stay sunk pointing towards the floor. (Fig c) PAUSE.

- Now repeat, pushing the heavy object away again, slowly and deliberately. PAUSE.

- Keep repeating this for a few moments, just enjoying the soft and relaxed, gentle stretching movement. WAIT.

- Now, as you continue the movement, begin to pay attention to your breathing again PAUSE, and every time you push the heavy object away, exhale slowly and continuously. PAUSE.

- As you relax and retract your arms, inhale slowly and continuously. PAUSE.

- Don't force your breathing, just allow the movement to flow with your breathing. PAUSE.

- Exhaling as you push away, and inhaling as you relax. PAUSE.

- Repeat this until it is comfortable. WAIT.

- Now, as you relax your arms and inhale, pay attention to your palms, and imagine you are inhaling into the centre of the palms. PAUSE.

- As you push again, exhale as before through pursed lips. PAUSE.

- Just enjoy this for as long as you are comfortable. PAUSE.

- Inhaling into the centre of the palms, PAUSE.

- Don't worry about whether you are doing it right or not, it is only a taster. WAIT.

- When you are ready, just slowly lower your arms to the side of your body, and breathe normally. PAUSE.

Who says I can't?

- If you feel a slight tingling or warmth in the palms, don't worry, it is perfectly normal and a nice feeling. PAUSE.

- Just stay in this position and breathe normally and gently for a few moments. WAIT.

- Now, I want you to move your arms around towards the front of the body again, but still allow them to just hang loosely, keeping the fingers and thumbs open. PAUSE.

- Now imagine having balloons tied to each wrist, just allow your wrists to begin slowly floating up in front of your body, with your arms comfortably extended and the fingers hanging loose until they are about chest height. (Fig e) PAUSE.

- Keep your arms comfortably extended away from you, but don't allow the elbows to lock. The movement is soft. PAUSE.

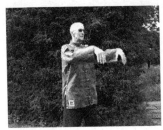
Fig e

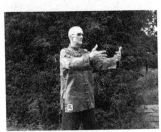
Fig f

Joe Lodge

- Now, as though you were throwing open your arms, but in very slow motion, turn your finger tips to face in towards each other so your left hand fingers are facing to your right and your right hand fingers are facing towards your left (Fig f), allow your palms to move away from each other as you open your arms slowly out towards the sides of your body, (Fig g) PAUSE.

- Do this gently until you feel the shoulder blades moving together. PAUSE.

- Enjoy the feeling of gently stretching, but don't let the shoulder blades touch. PAUSE.

- Now you should have your arms extended sideways, with your palms open and facing forwards. (Fig h) PAUSE.

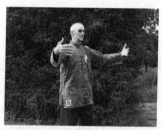
Fig g

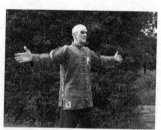
Fig h

- Now, just allow the palms to move back towards each other, arms still extended, until the palms are facing each other in front of the body again, about chest height and shoulder width apart. (Fig i) PAUSE.

Who says I can't?

- Now turn the palms to face down. (Fig j) PAUSE.

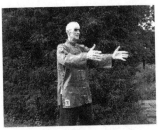
Fig i

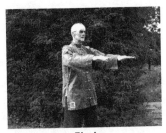
Fig j

- Now just allow the knees to bend and sink your body slightly just as though you were going to sit on the edge of a table. PAUSE.

- At the same time, bring the palms down towards the floor, still facing down, PAUSE, and then relax the wrists and allow the fingers to sink and face the floor. (Fig k) PAUSE.

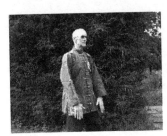
Fig k

- Now repeat the movements (Fig e-k) by raising the body a little, then the arms again, to chest height, PAUSE, slowly open the arms fully, PAUSE, then close the palms towards each other until they are shoulder width apart, turn them face down and sink. PAUSE.

- Repeat (Fig e-k) and allow the movement to become **slow, flowing and soft**. WAIT.

- Once you are comfortable with the movement, just continue, and then pay attention to your breathing. PAUSE.

- Try to inhale as you raise and open your arms, then exhale as you bring them together and lower them. PAUSE.

- If that is too difficult or you don't understand it, don't worry, just breathe naturally. Enjoy the feeling of gently opening the chest. WAIT.

- When you are ready to finish this movement, just allow the arms to settle at the side of the body again and relax, breathing normally. PAUSE

- Just stand in this position for a few moments and pay attention to your body and how good this feels. WAIT.

- To finish, just gently shake your arms and legs. If your palms tingle a little just rub them together, then shake them. This is normal. WAIT.

End – Well done

Who says I can't?

The first few movements were just simple relaxation movements to help your body, mind and breathing relax and coordinate. The last movement is known as 'Open the chest' and would normally be repeated eight times as part of a daily routine with seventeen other movements, known as Shibashi. There are many versions of this, and plenty of video demonstrations on the internet, especially on You Tube. Shibashi (18 Movements of Tai Chi Qi Gung) is a very simple set of movements and ideal for beginners. It can also be modified to be done while seated (good for recovery after exacerbations).

Tai Chi and Qi Gung (don't worry if you can't pronounce it!) have hundreds of different movements, all having slightly different effects on the energy system of the body, the one you have just tried is of interest to COPD patients as it helps to stimulate the lung meridian according to the Tai Chi classical masters. Of course doing all the eighteen movements together daily, helps to benefit all areas of the body (and mind).

I hope you enjoyed that little taster and maybe it will inspire you to find a local class and have a go.

It is an enjoyable little daily session anyway and should leave you feeling relaxed.

For me, Tai Chi has been the 'bedrock' of my life for the last fifteen years, helping me to maintain a healthy body and mind, and helping me to feel empowered to have some control over my own health beside the traditional health system. My daily Tai Chi is as natural as my breathing now!

Joe Lodge

Footnote – here are a few basic physical and mental benefits relevant to COPD:

- Improves posture over time, which allows the lungs to move more freely.

- Muscles remain more relaxed reducing the need for metabolic oxygen.

- More efficient movement over time, reducing effort and oxygen waste.

- Improves posture balance reducing the risk of falls with ageing.

- Improves the overall balance of the body. As we spend a whole lifetime being left or right handed and mal-adjusting our posture and movement to suit, much better use of balanced movement improves oxygen use.

- Gentle and controlled movement of all the body's joints encouraging synovial fluid lubrication and looseness of joints during ageing.

- Improved diaphragm and intercostal muscle strength and use during abdominal breathing.

- Relaxation window expands over a period, from the after effects of a session until it begins to spill into your whole day, even beginning with anticipation relaxation.

Who says I can't?

- Could also be recommended for patients partners as an ideal way to 'escape' and relax.

- Improves mindfulness, the ability to be aware of what you are doing at this moment in time without intrusive thoughts.

- Raises your spirits!

**"Bugs don't nest in a busy doorway"
Chinese proverb.**

Joe Lodge

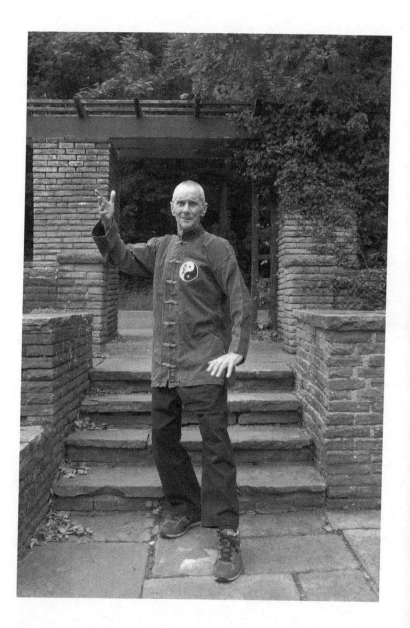

Who says I can't?

Complementary Therapies

There are many complementary therapies available to most people such as Reiki and Acupuncture. In my experience patients with long term conditions such as COPD are always interested in something that may provide a little more benefit to their daily life besides the normal medications that they use to manage their condition.

I find patients fall into three categories here, those that are open and self-motivated enough to give something a realistic trial and then adopt it or move on, those that are sceptical of everything unless administered by their doctor and those who are indifferent. If you are of the latter types then just leave complementary therapies alone.

I have tried Reiki, Acupuncture and Acupressure over the years with varying degrees of improvement but nothing that would be classed as significant. However, that does not mean that you would have the same results. I may not have given them a fair trial, I may have tried them at a time when my lungs were not in a good enough shape to respond. I may have tried a 'poor' practitioner.

Just for clarity I have noted my thoughts on each of these, but again remember that my experience is subjective, you may have a completely different experience.

Joe Lodge

Reiki – level 1

I did not try this specifically for my breathing, merely from my interest in relaxation techniques. It is a very pleasurable and relaxing session in which you basically just have to lie on a therapist's table while they perform various hand movements over areas of your body. If you enjoy internal feelings and energy work this is definitely worth a session. I would consider Reiki of possible benefit to anyone who has difficulty with relaxation or emotional difficulty in dealing with their COPD. It did not affect my breathing in any way.

Acupuncture

Whilst I consider acupuncture a serious form of therapy that aims directly to relieve the symptoms of COPD by the insertion of painless needles into various points around the body, stimulating the balance and smooth flow of the body's energy (chi), I did not find a significant improvement in my breathing although my chest did feel a lot looser. I possibly didn't give it a fair trial as it is rather expensive and requires a number of sessions. I believe my daily tai chi practice does the same thing in a more subtle manner over a period of time. Had I not practiced Tai Chi I would have probably had monthly acupuncture sessions. It is for you to try and decide if it provides you with any real or apparent benefit.

Who says I can't?

Acupressure

This is similar to acupuncture except the needles are replaced by the body's own massage tools like fingers, knuckles and joints. These are used in a similar manner to acupuncture, by massaging and stimulating various points on the body to help restore balance and flow of energy. The interesting thing here is that you can visit a therapist or, if you are able, you can easily learn the basics and self- administer this, which is the path I took. Again, I cannot report any significant improvement in my breathing. However, I have found it an increasingly interesting tool in a number of areas. While learning some simple points to massage I discovered one that appears to have resolved my 'foggy brain', which I have heard many COPD patients complain of. It is a feeling of not being quite 'in the present' and of being unable to think clearly, also one of the main reasons for me taking so long to write this book! Would this work for you? I don't know, but it does bring me to my main point about therapies which is the question you would have to answer:

Do you want to keep paying someone else to do something to you or do you want to learn how to do something yourself?

My personal approach is that I may pay for a taster session but I would always prefer to learn a technique for myself that I can administer as often as I like, when I like. This was one of my main reasons for taking up Tai Chi.

This was something I could learn and then 'practise' daily for myself.

My advice is that if it makes you feel good, then try it, there is never anything to lose by trying new experiences. Even the psychological benefit of feeling self-empowered is enough to justify it.

Of course the best therapy of all is – ACTIVITY

Supplements

There are many supplements on the market, all making some form of claim as to the benefits they may bring and I do try to keep abreast of what is available should a slot arise for a clinical trial in my laboratory (me!). While these things may be frowned on by your health provider they may have some positive effects on you, directly or indirectly. If you are smart enough to do your research first to determine if you think a supplement may be worth trying, and you are confident and sensible enough to plan a course of it then why not give it a try? It will at least help you feel that you have some personal control over your disease. Even if it's only a placebo effect, this is just as real as any other effect. If it helps you breathe better, then it does.

I try to use the internet for the 'Cloud Laboratory' feedback, which means that if so many people around the world report that something has benefited them,

Who says I can't?

then, even knowing that a percentage would be waffle or false promotion, it is worth investigating whether it could benefit me. Although I have taken many supplements, as I showed during my 'Cure Trial' mentioned earlier, I only mention a couple of supplements in this section as these serve to illustrate my approach and results. Of course you should check with your health provider that any supplement won't interact with your current medication.

While mainstream medicine is good for treating and managing your COPD and exacerbations, as mentioned with therapies, many people feel they want to try more to improve their quality of life and may decide to try alternative medicines or supplements. You may have heard for instance, that Oxy Moxy (a seaweed derivative), can increase the amount of oxygen carried in the blood which could help improve your daily level of breathlessness. There are many things advertised that may or may not work for you. Should you try them? If you are adventurous enough to try different things there are, in my experience, a few simple trial rules to follow:

1. **Don't expect instant results**
   Most alternative medicines, supplements and therapies work on a more natural, subtle level than western medicine, so results may take some time and may not be dramatic. Bearing in mind that you have probably had a chronic illness for years, expecting overnight changes is not realistic, but not impossible either.

2. **Don't expect dramatic results**
It may be that over a period of time you get a subtle improvement in your daily breathing which does not appear significant, but if it is due to the supplement or therapy, then adding this to the things that are good for you may make all the difference. I have said many times that if I could just improve my breathing by a few percent it would make all the difference.

3. **Try them for a realistic time period**
My personal guideline on this is twelve weeks. I know many people who have said, "Oh I tried a couple of sessions of that, didn't do anything for me". Hold on, you didn't even give it a chance! It may take time to build to a level where it starts to make a difference. It may be that by keeping a diary of the small improvements (if there are any) which you can compare using your daily markers such as dressing or walking (anything you do repeatedly and daily) helps you to make an informed judgement of any improvement. In my experience I generally notice a difference within days but sometimes it has taken a couple of weeks. (Perhaps I'm just a sensitive, city boy?)

4. **Decide for yourself if you are going to try something**
Don't be put off by friends or relatives who say it's a load of rubbish or just a placebo effect. The FACT is – IT DOESN'T MATTER! All that matters is

Who says I can't?

whether or not it makes any difference to YOU. Some people swear by paracetamol, others by ibuprofen. We are all different and cannot always predict what will work for each other.

The bottom line is that the placebo effect is very real and can be used to your advantage, if you perceive and believe that something is benefiting you. Your body's inert abilities are really amazing!

The other positive effect of trying supplements (or therapies) is that you start to pay more attention to your body and how it feels and reacts on a daily basis at a subtle level. This is a great help to improve your self-monitoring skills. Be adventurous if you are confident to try things, ask for your partner's or family's support if you are not sure, but don't just dismiss ANYTHING, it could be just what works for you. Trying new things is always interesting and can help you feel more empowered that you are not solely reliant on 'the system' to manage your illness, but able to make small improvements yourself.

The Oxy Moxy I referred to above is available on the internet. As it is supposed to work almost immediately (I understand airline pilots may use it to help reduce jet lag) I initially thought I would try it before exercise or my Tai Chi classes to see if it made any difference. It didn't. Then I got to thinking that it could be more subtle, so I tried it on a regular basis during normal days and noticed a definite difference to my resting breath over a period of time. As I had not made any other changes or introduced any other supplements, I had to conclude the improvement was down to the Oxy Moxy. It is rather expensive however, so I decided the subtle benefit didn't justify the cost. Maybe it would be different for you.

If you do decide that you should try a supplement or make adjustments to dosages of supplements (as they are not always very clear), remember the Golden Rule of clinical trials, **only make one change at a time**, and use the lowest dose that provides the desired effect. I found that by keeping a diary, as though I was doing a clinical trial, allowed me to check back and confirm that I did actually see an improvement. I would also recommend from experience that you **don't allow yourself to become dependent on any supplements or alternative medicines and therapies**. If they do help, carry them on for a maximum of twelve weeks, then give your body a rest and see if you need to return to them or whether your body has recovered from that need. Don't stay on anything blindly just because it worked initially.

Colloidal Silver

Another example for me is Colloidal Silver, which, although not recognised as a supplement, has in my view dramatically reduced my hospital visits due to exacerbations. I used to be in hospital every winter with pneumonia, almost guaranteed! Since taking a daily background dose of Colloidal Silver through the winter months, I have not been admitted for this and have actually made it through winter without my obligatory

Who says I can't?

'hospital holiday'. I used to have a bag packed ready for hospital just in case, as it happened that often, but now I don't bother because it has become a rarity. I did need to find the correct dose, as many supplements do not come with guidelines and unless you are methodical in your approach to this I would recommend you leave well alone. My dose of Colloidal Silver was one teaspoon a day between August and March, then I would give my body a rest during summer months when infections are less likely.

If I felt an infection coming on (breathlessness, green phlegm and temperature) I would increase this to three teaspoons a day. I have not suffered any side effects from this.

I discovered it on the internet while researching the effectiveness of antibiotics, which, as you probably are aware, are sometimes targeted at a very narrow range of bacteria and sometimes broad spectrum, which cover a number of bacteria and may be given when the exact cause of infection isn't known. I was looking for something natural that could also combat viral infections. Let me repeat that colloidal silver is advertised and sold on the internet, but it is not approved for sale as a medicine or food supplement (in the EU). The claim made by the silver manufacturers is that silver has been laboratory tested and shown to kill 650 known bacteria, viral and fungal pathogens (foreign cells that invade the body). The obvious question is, "If this is true, why on earth isn't it used by the heath authorities?" I believe there are two main reasons, the first being that a certain individual ingested large quantities of silver (not colloidal silver) and this caused an irreversible change of skin colour to a blueish grey colour. This was taken as a warning not to use it. I do not know of any other recorded problem or incident to date. Prior to the discovery of penicillin, it was known that silver could help fight 'germs' and some people would lick a silver teaspoon when they were ill.

Sources on the internet state that the real reason that silver is not used by the health providers is that they can only use clinically trialled and proven medicines, which is, of course, the correct approach for them. So in the UK, this would have to be passed by NICE (National Institution for Clinical Excellence) which would involve years of clinical trials. Who would fund this research? Much research is done by, or on behalf of, and funded by the pharmaceutical industry. Now let's think about this. Silver is a natural metal so can't be patented. Water also cannot be patented. So if colloidal silver was tested, proven and accepted by the health authorities, would the pharmaceutical industry lose millions in revenue? If, on the other hand, they fund research into medicines that will 'manage' your symptoms, and ensure you live for as long as possible...a patient cured is a customer lost...

As ingesting any form of metal over a period of time is very much frowned on by the medical authorities, I am not in any way recommending that you try it. I evaluate

Who says I can't?

and take full responsibility for any trials I conduct and I include mention of it here for completeness.

Salt Pipe

This is not a supplement but an aid to patients with COPD and, I believe, well worth a mention. Years ago (1843), a doctor in a village in Poland realised that the local population that worked in the nearby salt mine never suffered with respiratory problems. After some investigation he found that inhaling the salty air for even a short period each day, was beneficial in preventing respiratory issues and he produced a book on the subject. This information was only developed further in Hungary in 2002 when the salt pipe was born. This is just a ceramic pot containing a quantity of salt crystals. There is a grilled bottom to allow air flow across the crystals and through a mouthpiece. Breathing through this for just twenty minutes daily is reported to both reduce inflammation and infection in the lungs and helps to break up the sticky mucous that infections are so fond of!

Again I only tend to use this through the winter months which is just my personal preference. The useful thing is also that the twenty minutes can be split over the day, and as I lead such a busy life I am able to do five minutes in the morning and fifteen minutes in the evening (most days). The salt pipe is readily available on the internet and I believe is also being viewed seriously by mainstream health providers.

I have over the years tried many more supplements but none of these provided me with any significant improvements, indeed some had some unpleasant side effects. It is up to you the reader to decide if you want to try these things and I hope my experience and tips are at least helpful. **There is still no doubt though, the best supplement by far is ACTIVITY!**

The Other Passion

Okay, with COPD, your love life may slowly turn from Fifty Shades of Grey to Gone with the Wind (or is that came?). Obviously, sex requires extra oxygen and when your lungs don't come up with the goods any more, then your body may show signs of distress. Going at it like rabbits and then having to stop because you are gasping for air and look like you are about to burst, will leave you both frustrated and your partner worrying that you are going to have a heart attack! Go easy on yourself. If you are lucky to have a long term partner and you had a good sex life before your diagnosis, you may well both adapt as you deteriorate by taking things gentler and more loving.

If your partner has a high sex drive then you need to talk openly and frankly, there are many smart ways to enjoy sex and please each other without having to burst your lungs. If you do exercise regularly and have not been diagnosed with any greater risk of heart failure than expected for your age, then you are extremely unlikely to have a heart attack during sex and frankly, if you do,

Who says I can't?

while it may be very inconsiderate to your partner, can you think of a better way to go? Keep sex light hearted, talk openly and just do whatever it is you can to please each other. My personal experience of sex with emphysema is...Doh! Just when I am pouring my heart out, my mind goes blank! Yeah right! Did you really think I was going to go that far? Ha! You couldn't handle it!

Reflections

As I write this book it is fifteen years since I was diagnosed with emphysema. Looking back, I have to ask myself, "Could I have done anything different or better that would have slowed my rate of decline?" The answer is a simple 'yes'. Everyone's lung function has a natural slow rate of decline as the decades roll by. After my initial diagnosis aged forty five, my equivalent lung age was one hundred and thirteen! I don't know or care to know what it is now. The main observation I have made over this period is that the decline in my lung function didn't occur gradually, it happened in steps, each time I had a bad exacerbation, usually Pneumonia.

No doubt, in the background I had the natural and very slow decline, but this was masked by the Pneumonia steps. Whenever I eventually recovered, sometimes after a couple of weeks but commonly up to twelve or more weeks, I had definitely not recovered to the same level of breathing as before. As the years have passed it has taken longer to recover each time and after my last really bad episode it took nearly six months to recover to a reasonable level again. After say two months, it is all too easy to fall into the mind set of 'this is it now, I am not going to recover any further'. Don't fall for that one, always believe that you will keep on recovering and eat, sleep and exercise as well as you can along the way. Never give up hope. I am naturally positive but there have been a number of times when even I have fallen into this trap and started to resign myself to a very poor outlook, only to find a couple of weeks later that my breathing has improved. I don't know of any miracles or short cuts to recovery, only patience and faith in your own body's amazing abilities of recovery.

"Never say die till you're dead!" (Gentle version – "Never give up")

So, "What could I have done better?" I know that I analyse things too much and there are many occasions where I have been trying to determine whether I have a chest infection coming on or whether it is just a bad spell. I was often wrong and would always leave it too long before seeking help, by which time I would normally take a really bad turn and end up in hospital. Had I gone straight to the surgery at the early symptoms or, as now, had I started taking antibiotics straight away, I am convinced I would have caught and cured the Pneumonia earlier with a lot less permanent damage. I would often

Who says I can't?

get caught out when feeling ill during the week, by thinking I'll see how it goes over the weekend, only to find by Sunday I needed an ambulance.

So my advice is simple, and the single most important thing I have to say in this whole book is, if you can have standby antibiotics in the home, as I do now, then get them and use them at the first sign of a chest infection. If not, then visit your healthcare provider as soon as you start to have symptoms of a chest infection...And stay active!

Of course, prevention is better than cure. I know there were times when I hadn't eaten well for a week or two, particularly if we had been away from home and living on fast foods too often. That was a mistake I won't repeat. It is surprising how weak your immune system can become with emphysema. Also, I wish I had discovered the Colloidal Silver and Salt pipe in my early emphysema days. I know there is no scientific evidence that they will prevent infection but I believe they have helped me. Whether it is the placebo effect or not I could not care less. You must discover what works best for you and take some responsibility for your health.

I do try to avoid public transport, but not the cinema, theatre or shops, I just get on with life and do not wrap myself in cotton wool. Maybe sometimes I get it wrong but at least I am living, not just coping!

I believe my approach to staying active has helped me lead a normal life, albeit a bit slower, and I often meet healthy people who haven't done half the things I have. I guess healthy people can afford the luxury of complacency. Don't fall for that one! I know my biggest mistake has almost always been to 'battle on' and delay seeking help.

I know that over the next few years I will have to face new challenges. For how long will I be able to keep working? How long before I need home oxygen? Is it time to start planning my funeral?

Life continuously evolves and I must evolve with it and devise new solutions to new challenges as they arise. I focus on living, not on COPD.

Anyway, here I am, fifteen years on, still working and still a lone parent, although I'm pleased to say that as I finish writing this book, my daughter has just got her place confirmed at university and has now left home. "Oh dear, life will be so quiet and I'm going to miss her so much. "Whatever will I do with my free time now?"..."Party time!...Where's my little black book?"...

Living with a 'duffer' – my daughter's perspective

As I draw towards the end of this book, I realise that while I have tried to give you an insight into how COPD may affect you and your loved ones and hopefully given you some tips on how to manage your illness better, I feel that I don't really know how my illness has affected my daughter. At nineteen (now) she has only really

Who says I can't?

known me with emphysema and the way of life that entails, so I thought it would be fitting to ask my daughter to write a chapter for you telling her view on how my illness has affected her and her thoughts on the matter. Maybe this would help with your loved ones understanding of your COPD from a different angle.

I have tried to do my best as a parent and no doubt, some of my drive comes from being a lone parent with no help and having the need to carry on even when it was too hard. I have always tried to be independent and not rely on anyone else for help, but there have been times when my daughter has kept the home running. I have always told her I do not want her to become my carer. And that will always be the case. I would rather go into a care home than to become a burden and stop her from spreading her wings. I think it has brought us very close on a deep level, as we have shared many good times and bad. She has had her own share of issues to deal with as well as putting up with the 'duffer'.

She has not read my book as she writes her chapter and I have decided that I will not edit or comment on her words, as I owe it to her and you, the reader, to make sure I don't influence her words in any way, so you get a genuine account. Whether I thank her afterwards or not is another matter, but then I have to be careful what I say don't I, as she may be the one choosing my care home one day...

Joe Lodge

Kim's Words

The only way I can describe how it is to live with my dad is it's like having 'second-hand' emphysema. I obviously don't have the physical symptoms that the illness entails, but when you live with someone who's physically ill, you experience the same ups and downs as them, you get to see how it effects what would be a 'regular' life, how things change, how the struggle kicks in. Believe me, when you're a healthy person, it can be hilariously gross to see the symptoms of emphysema in all their glory, but you have to take it in your stride, and hold on to the fact that there are good days, not just bad ones.

When I think about it, I've been lucky in the sense that I was only about 4 years old when my dad got emphysema, so I've never really known any different, but I can't imagine how difficult it must be to see a healthy person transition into this. One thing I do know though, is that kids are resilient, and yes, they will ask a lot of questions and stare, but they'll just get on with life, probably not knowing that anything's even wrong. My earliest memory of actually realising that there was something wrong with my dad was when I was about 5 and I was perplexed as to why he couldn't chase me round the house playing tag, but we got past that problem by switching to computer games instead!

I think my 'issues' with emphysema only kicked in when I was a typical pre-teen, angry at the world and embarrassed by everything. The question of 'why me?'

Who says I can't?

always used to bother me, and I know that it seems selfish because I wasn't the person who was actually ill. Over time you realise that people with emphysema can't just walk away from it, but everyone close to them can. You do witness the breakdown of relationships and friendships, but however harsh it seems, you have to be reasonable and understand that is does have a great emotional toll on second-hand sufferers and that sometimes it's just too much. For me, no matter how tough things got, I never had the option to walk away. I was young and my dad was the only person there for me. I've never been labelled as a 'carer', but it is so unbelievably difficult to be the main support for someone who is ill. It feels like a difficult line to cross to be labelled as a carer and you feel unjustified, like there's always someone else out there who's worse off than you.

I managed to hide what was going on at home, whether it was the right thing to do or not, all the way through school and up until the 3rd year of college. It was the start of a new academic year and my dad had just been hospitalised with pneumonia again. I coped well at home, but after a few days my emotional barrier just came tumbling down and I ended up running to my course leader and crumpled up into a ball on the floor, crying hysterically. Telling someone what was going off and having to explain everything (especially when people are so perplexed about how my dad still manages to work full time) was one of the most difficult things I've ever done, and it's probably one of the only things that I struggle to talk to people about. Sharing everything with someone felt so painful at the time, but the relief afterwards was immense and I do sort of regret that I'd not done it earlier.

I'm an independent person and hate people fussing over me, but I really do have to hand it to the people who taught me at college. After discovering all of this, they managed to step back and not get too involved, whilst they still always made sure I was coping okay and I knew that I could talk to them whenever the second-hand illness was making me have a bad day. They did arrange for me to go to a young carers group, but as I mentioned earlier, even after sharing everything with someone, I still felt unjustified.

Looking back, my advice to anyone else in a similar situation would be to go for it. No one has a right to judge or label whether you're having to care for someone and deal with the emotional side of an illness, and if you feel like it's affecting you and you need to get it all off your chest and talk to people who actually understand what it's like, because if it makes you feel better, then it's clearly the right thing to do, regardless of what anyone else thinks.

I feel like a big moment for my dad was getting the supplementary oxygen. He's a proud man, and he would never admit it, but it embarrassed him and he became uncharacteristically self-conscious. People stare, especially kids, but it's just human nature and I doubt anyone means to cause any hurt. Even I still take a second look at people with oxygen on even though I live with someone who has it!

Who says I can't?

The option of going to university was something that naturally cropped up in my life quite recently and obviously I did want to go, but I was scared of leaving my dad. I know the last thing he wanted to do was to stop me from moving on in life, but because of how he is and how much of a role I've previously played in his care when he's been badly, I decided to stay in my home town so that I could be there for him, as well as other medical reasons of my own.

Going on to being morbid, whether you like it or not, everyone around you is slowly dying. The problem with being close to someone who is ill is that the situation is a little more obvious, but you just have to accept it and take each day as it comes, no matter how painful it is. You can feel sorry for yourself and wallow in sadness all you like, but it doesn't do anything to change the situation. I did want to go to universities in different cities, but what I wanted more and still want, is to be here for if my dad needs me and enjoy the time we've got left together, whether that be 4 years or 14!

Before I moved into student accommodation, I did worry loads about who was going to be there in emergencies, who would help to clean, who was going to call the ambulance when needed, etc., but you have to put yourself first sometimes and get on with your own life, even if both of you feel bad about it, it's something that simply has to happen. I do sit here and wonder whether he's okay, how his SATs are, whether he's relying on oxygen a lot, etc., but I have to control those thoughts and trust that if he needs me, he knows I'm there. I do however know that my dad's a sneaky one for not telling people when he's been hospitalised, and he will be in big trouble with me if I find out he's not told me at some point!

In summary, if you're going through this as whatever relation to a patient at whatever age, just hold on in there. It is challenging, you can't predict how things will be, and you are required to have a lot of patience. The only thing that will make your position better is acceptance. Yes, it sucks, but unfortunately you can't change it. Be there through the bad times, laugh at the good times, and most importantly, don't forget to live your own life and look after yourself!

All I really have to say is thank you dad. Thank you for putting up with me and doing an outstanding job of raising me and shaping me into the adult I have become today, despite all your own problems and troubles.

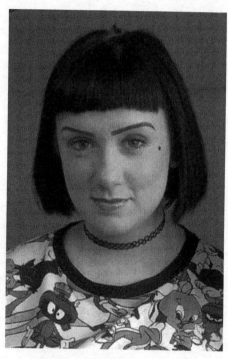

Kimberley Lodge

Part 3 Summary

- Physically and mentally, take responsibility for your general, daily health.

- Do everything with PASSION!

- Most tasks can be broken down into smaller and smaller chunks until they become manageable.

- Try to do everything yourself, just in a different way.

- Join a fun exercise class.

- Adapt, improvise and overcome – don't see obstacles, see challenges!

- The Placebo Effect is real – if something makes you feel or breathe better, use it!

- Be kind to your heart.

- Always have standby antibiotics.

- Review everything in your life and set a goal.

So what should

I do next?

Health Professionals

Keep doing what you do best, helping us to manage our COPD and picking us up when we get it wrong or it all gets too much for us, but also see that it's not just a long slippery slope of decline. Tell patients and their partners that once they get to grips with a different lifestyle they can achieve amazing things and enjoy life again, just in a new way. Tell them of examples like mine, there is nothing more reassuring than knowing that someone with a lower FEV1% predicted than yours can actually do exciting things and live life to the full in their own way. Above all, tell them this with genuine enthusiasm. Ask your patients for photos of their achievements to put on your wall as a reminder to yourself and an inspiration to all your patients of what they can actually do. Look at the crazes on You Tube, we have extreme ironing, extreme marriages, why not extreme COPD?! Make the tee shirt, create the movie, who knows what you can do until you try?! Wind them up and send them off looking for new ways to tackle life, full of hope and inspiration!

Friends

Do what good friends naturally do, just be there. We do want to do things and share experiences with you, we just worry that if we make plans, we will often let you down on the day, so we may shy off taking up any offers and you may feel you are helping by not offering and putting us in that position. Nah! Just carry on asking us to go to the pub, country or whatever and if we have a bad 'air' day and can't, just give us a light hearted, sarcastic, reminder of what we are missing and we'll look forward to the next time.

Family

You are our lifeline, the people we need to help us when we just can't manage. You are the ones who see COPD in its raw state. You may have fallen into the trap of becoming our carer. The best thing I could ask of you is to sit down with us and discuss what you have read in this book and talk openly and honestly about how our illness has affected you. About the things you do for us. Review everything, from the shopping you collect for us to painting the garden fence and see if we could find new and exciting ways to tackle things. Talk about experiences we can share together, a day in the park or country, maybe at the coast. Brainstorm smart ways to do things that you have previously had to stop because of our illness. Be enthusiastic with us. We can do more. Keep it light hearted with that magic ingredient of a dash of sarcasm, it keeps everyone smiling, and you always look forward to seeing someone who makes you smile, don't you?

If you have young children just be aware if they have any bugs before you visit and make allowances, but don't

Who says I can't?

keep them away. Playing with young children is a great distraction and it's easy to forget your own troubles in their company. They are also good at thinking outside the box, so let them join in brainstorming how you are going to paint that fence or go extreme mobility scooting.

Partners

I really hope my book helps you to understand us a little better and helps to open an honest reappraisal of how you feel about our illness and the way it has affected your life.

The very first thing you should discuss is not me, but you! Tell me one thing that you have been missing or longing to do for years and never had the opportunity. Now you have. Let's find a way between us that allows you to start doing that one thing at least once a week without any guilt, worry or strings. Do it. We will both feel so much better, and you will find a subconscious weight lifted from you and come back with a smile and a fresh spirit, ready to help me find new ways of tackling things. It doesn't have to be dramatic, maybe you have cooked all the meals since I was diagnosed to try to save me the exertion. Well how about getting the cookbook out and planning a meal to cook together? We could shop for the ingredients and I would get a little exercise. I could sit and peel potatoes or spin salad while you do the strenuous bit with all the pots and pans.

Joe Lodge

The main point is that we do something together rather than you doing something for me. Talk about it. Talk about the things we both used to enjoy doing together and see if there are new ways to allow us to at least recapture some of that magic, or even new things we have never thought of. Plan to have some exciting times together. Don't forget plan B though, should it all go wrong on the day. Keep it light hearted with a dash of wicked sarcasm and we all end up smiling no matter what! Thanks for being there. Good luck.

You

You are the one person who is going to make the most difference to the rest of your life!

What should you do now? If you are still a smoker, then get smart and prepare a battle plan involving as many different strategies as you can and just imagine yourself as a non-smoker, enjoying the fresh air and freedom in the country.

Define yourself. I am not a COPD patient who manages as well as possible, I am Joe, I have a job, I am a parent, I have lots of hobbies and interests, hopes and dreams, and yes, I do have COPD, which can limit my abilities, but I just get on with life and deal with it when necessary. Who are you? How do you define yourself? How would you like to define yourself?

Very early on in the book, I mentioned a magic bullet. Well there really is one, you can find it in the nearest mirror!

Who says I can't?

Complete the Life Review Checklist I have added at the end of the book (Appendix A), to help you evaluate where you are now in terms of general activity and to help you decide how you could improve on that. Who knows, maybe together we can change the statistics on COPD patients!

Make a list now of all the things you used to enjoy doing but have had to give up. Think about new ways to micro manage them. Ask your family and friends to help. Make a list of things you always wanted to do or need to do and have never got started. Bring some excitement into your life, always have something 'on the boil' that you look forward to.

Make sure you have antibiotics on hand to catch any bacteria that sneak up on you.

Eat well, rest well, exercise well and play well.

Each time you wake up remind yourself, **today is a brand new day!** How exciting is that? What are you going to do with it?

STAY ACTIVE!

Oh, I nearly forgot, what about my next challenge?...hmmm...How many steps does the Eiffel Tower have?

The End?...

Appendix A – Life Review Checklist

To help you think about what you can do next, I have created a simple check list below of general living activities that you may do daily or periodically. Some don't appear immediately to be an activity until you really think about them. The benefit of lots of little activities is cumulative, try them.

Looking at the Activity column, add a Score against each one based on your current life and the following key:

> 2 points = I do this myself
> 1 point = I do this with assistance
> 0 points = someone does this for me OR
> I do not do this at all

Then add your score. As there are 50 activities, the maximum score achievable would be 100, so anything you score below this will give you a percentage (i.e. if you score a total of 71, this is 71/100 = 71%)

Now look at each Activity again and think about what you could do differently to improve the score and then mark the figure in the New Score column. Now you can see what your improvement can be if you make a little effort.

OR you can just make up your own list now...GOOD LUCK!

Joe Lodge

Activity	Score	How can I improve this?	New Score
Get out of bed			
Get dressed			
Make a bed			
Have wash/shower/bath			
Shave or put on make-up			
Brush teeth (own or not!)			
Prepare breakfast			
Morning walk or exercise			
Prepare lunch			
Go to work (paid or not)			
Evening walk or exercise			
Prepare evening meal			
Wash dishes/cutlery			
Make drink for partner			
Vacuum a carpet			
Sweep a floor			
Mop a floor			
Hang washing out			
Put rubbish out			
Iron clothes			
Clean lower windows			
Mow the lawn			
Trim hedge			

Who says I can't?

Activity	Score	How can I improve this?	New Score
Weed a border			
Pot some flowers			
Use watering can			
Walk to local shop			
Carry shopping bags			
Drive a car			
Wash a car			
Put fuel in a car			
Avoid disabled parking			
Walk for 30 minutes			
Visit supermarket			
Push shopping trolley			
Put shopping away			
Visit family or friends			
Attend activity or class			
Make someone laugh			
Send partner out for night			
Try new activity			
Try new food			
Assist someone worse off			
Collect own meds			
Splash in a puddle			
Visit your town centre			

Joe Lodge

Activity	Score	How can I improve this?	New Score
Do something spontaneous			
ADD YOUR OWN			
1.			
2.			
3.			
Phew! Who needs a gym?			

Appendix B – Cure Trial Log

Date	10/12/12	Notes
Day	**Mon**	
Medications	Ventolin 100ug inhaler Atrovent 20ug inhaler Seretide 500 Acuhaler Antibiotic Co-Amoxiclav	2 puffs 4 x daily 2 puffs 4 x daily 1 puff 2 x daily 1 tablet 3 x daily
Breakfast	USN IGF Pure Protein mix (0.6g) + porridge oats (12g) + Warburtons wholemeal toast (0.9g) + butter (clover)	1 x scoop +75ml water +150ml soya milk+ 5ml flax oil + ½ banana + 1 drop Vitamin A supplement (5000iu) 1 slice
Lunch	Homemade Romain salad + 3 slices ham + 2 slices above wholemeal bread & butter (1.8g)	3 Romaine leaves + portion of Sainsbury Rainbow salad
Tea	Grilled burger(0.4g) + Romaine salad and oven fries (1.0g)	(okay, it's still a transition!)
Supper	Peanut butter sandwich on wholemeal bread	Felt good after this
Snacks	Nature valley oats & honey crunchy bar (5.6g)	
Drinks	Tea + soya milk Water	
Objective	Morning Tai Chi was good. Started to remove refined sugar from diet. No more in tea (about 8-10 tsps per day.) No more biscuits (about 6-8 per day ....a work institution!)	Had bought Actimel probiotics but I think if I am taking anitibiotics as well this is just going to waste their time, they need to aim for the bad guys. They can wait till antib's finished.
Subjective	Gone from despising tea without sugar to accepting it so can look forward to cuppa again.	Couldn't finish burger or fries but salad was moreish...is my body telling me something?

Joe Lodge

Date	13/12/12	Notes
Day	**Thur**	
Medications	Ventolin 100ug inhaler Atrovent 20ug inhaler Seretide 500 Acuhaler	2 puffs 4 x daily 2 puffs 4 x daily 2 x puff daily
Supplements	Actimel probiotic Vitamin A	
Breakfast	USN IGF Pure Protein mix (0.6g) + porridge oats (12g) + Warburtons wholemeal toast (0.9g) + butter (clover)	1 x scoop +75ml water +150ml soya milk+ 5ml flax oil + ½ banana + 1 drop Vitamin A supplement (5000iu) 1 slice
Lunch	Homemade Romain salad ¼ small pork pie (1g) 2 x hard boiled eggs + 1 slice above wholemeal bread & butter (0.9g)	3 Romaine leaves + portion of Sainsbury Classic salad
Tea	2 Bacon 1 sausage Baked beans (3g!)+ 1/2grilled tomato	Easier tea for Tai Chi class
Supper	Small piece cheese and small piece pork pie	
Snacks	Peanut butter sandwich (2)	
Drinks	Tea with soya milk / water /glass of rose wine	
Objective	Sats 96-98 at rest ! Walked round Sainsburys without zimmerframe (trolley) first time for year(s)?	Slightly less time to catch breath after getting in car and washing pots.
Subjective	Generally feel breathing has improved. Have coughed more mucus up than usual (none) maybe sugar reduction is allowing accumulated rubbish to clear from lungs.	It's only the first transition week to going sugar free although it's almost impossible to buy anything without some sugar.

Who says I can't?

Date	16/12/12	Notes
Day	Mon	
Medications	Ventolin 100ug inhaler Atrovent 20ug inhaler Seretide 500 Acuhaler Co Amoxiclav	2 puffs 4 x daily 2 puffs 4 x daily 2 puffs daily 3 tablets daily
Supplements	Actimel probiotic NAC 600mg capsule	
Breakfast	USN IGF Pure Protein mix (0.6g) + porridge oats (12g) + Warburtons wholemeal toast (0.9g) + butter (clover)	1 x scoop +75ml water +150ml soya milk+ 5ml flax oil + ½ banana 1 slice
Lunch	Homemade Romain salad + corned beef + 1 slice wholemeal bread (1.8g)	3 Romaine leaves + portion of Sainsbury Classic salad
Tea	Beefburger with caramelised onions+ steamed mixed vegetables+gravy	
Supper	Pork pie and cheese	
Snacks	2 x digestive biscuits	
Drinks	Tea with soya milk / water	
Objective	Decided to stop Vitamin A supplement today for a week. I feel like I have background headache which can be a sign of too much. Supplement is 5000IU + about 2000IU from breakfast shake+ daily from Romain lettuce I am probably on safe ceiling of 10000IU so will try 3 weeks on 1 week off as it stores in the liver.	As I am still coughing green phlegm and breathing not so good I have started another course of antibiotics to clear. When these are finished I will move onto supplement of Proteolytic Enzyme and Beta Glucan 1.3/1.6 to achieve same end of stripping pathogen protein coat and destroying pathogen.
Subjective		

Joe Lodge

Date	17/12/12	Notes
Day	**Tue**	
Medications	Ventolin 100ug inhaler Atrovent 20ug inhaler Seretide 500 Acuhaler Co Amoxiclav	2 puffs 4 x daily 2 puffs 4 x daily 2 puffs daily 3 tablets daily
Supplements	Actimel probiotic NAC 600mg capsule	In between antibiotic
Breakfast	USN IGF Pure Protein mix (0.6g) + porridge oats (12g) + Warburtons wholemeal toast (0.9g) + butter (clover)	1 x scoop +75ml water +150ml soya milk+ 5ml flax oil + ½ banana 1 slice
Lunch	Homemade Romain salad + corned beef	3 Romaine leaves + portion of Sainsbury Classic salad
Tea	½ a sirloin steak fried + a few oven bake fries + romain lettuce	
Supper	Pork pie + chees	
Snacks	Protein shake 2 x scoops + 150ml water + 150ml soya milk	Helped stop hunger
Drinks	Tea with soya milk / water	
Objective	Was right about Vitamin A headache cleared today.	As I have to gradually remove all sugar realised my porridge oats and banana had to go. So just protein shakes from now on.
Subjective	No changes...feeling hungry a lot so changing things round.	

About the Author

Joe has always been keen to pass his knowledge and experience on to others, whether in electronics or Tai Chi, qualifying as an adult education teacher with the opportunity to teach in college. However, as his COPD was progressing, his career path had to change to allow him to continue working but in an office environment as service manager for an electronics company, which was mentally challenging but physically manageable. He also attended the COPD Pulmonary Rehabilitation classes and participated in the NHS Expert Patient Programme.

Joe has learned to adapt his problem solving skills gained over forty years as an electronics engineer to overcome the many challenges of living with a progressive disease like COPD. Now he hopes to use those skills to help fellow COPD patients with inspiration and ideas through *Who Says I Can't? A Guide to Living Well with COPD*, his first book. He believes patients can do so much more to help themselves when inspired by another patient who has 'been there'.

Born and raised in South London, he left home at an early age to begin life's adventures, finally settling in Sheffield. His later years have been spent not only coping with the difficulties of COPD but also those of being a lone parent. Joe will continue to work as long as is physically possible during which time he would also like to spend more time writing about the realities of his disease progression and the new challenges he will have to face in the coming years.

Made in the USA
Charleston, SC
09 January 2016